Acknowledgments

I'm grateful to Dr. Michael Myers and Kathleen Border, R.D., for their help on some technical items. I wish to thank my editor, Michele Spence, for the time and effort she put into this work and for her patience with me. Thanks also to my reader, Maureen Leupold, and to my editor as well, for keeping me accurate.

Cover photograph by Tony Craddock/Tony Stone Images

FIRST EDITION

ISBN 0-8220-5330-6

CONTENTS

CONTENTS

CONTENTS

CONTENTS

CONTENTS

CONTENTS

CONTENTS

The **science of human nutrition,** like any other natural science, is an organized study of a natural phenomenon. In this case, the natural phenomenon is the role of food in the growth, development, and maintenance of the human body.

In general, sciences themselves are constantly growing and developing, the inevitable result of new knowledge being added to the field. Ongoing research, including laboratory studies with animals and medical studies on human subjects, is the source of the new knowledge, which often contradicts what is "known" about a subject. For example, several years ago, it was "common knowledge" that sugar was responsible for hyperactive behavior in children. However, as more research was conducted into the subject, it was found that this common knowledge was, frankly, wrong. Over the past 140 years or so, much of the common knowledge of human nutrition has been enhanced, modified, and in many instances disproved.

Unfortunately, as knowledge has advanced, so has myth and misinformation. Everybody has heard some of these, such as that eating protein promotes muscle development or that taking massive doses of vitamin E cures male pattern baldness. Where such ideas originate is, at best, out of wishful thinking and, at worst, out of deliberate deception to take advantage of human gullibility.

Nutrition scientists, medical doctors, physiologists, and **biochemists** conduct the research to develop knowledge. **Dieticians** are the practitioners who apply the knowledge.

Some History

Early in human history, food was procured by **hunting** and **gathering.** Hunting, the quest for meat, was sometimes successful and sometimes not. When it was, our ancestors ate well. Gathering was probably more consistently successful, and it provided fruits, vegetables, sometimes grains like wild rice, eggs, and possibly even meat in the form of small animals like insects or frogs. When food was abundant, people feasted and gained weight. However, food was not always abundant. In some parts of the world, severe winters meant seasonal periods of hunger, and those individuals who had not succeeded in storing enough food in the form of fat probably starved. In other parts of the world, prolonged dry seasons, in their own way as difficult as winters, often had to be endured. In addition to such periodic stresses, occasional natural disasters such as severe drought or floods could also mean instances of hunger. With such conditions, early humans may have experienced frequent disease, high infant mortality, and low fertility.

With the advent of **agriculture,** food availability probably became more assured. Episodic starvation no doubt continued, but it was more likely because of environmental disasters such as plagues of pests and extremely severe weather than seasonal changes. In addition, people learned something about **food preservation.** Practices like drying, pickling, and salting came about for that purpose. Additives were put in foods to keep them from spoiling. (The spices traded for by Europeans earlier in this millennium were not purchased for their enhancement of food flavors; they were used to keep foods edible. The spices tended to inhibit organisms that caused food spoilage.) Not all of the foods our ancestors gathered were suitable for cultivation, just as not all of the animals they hunted were suitable for domestication. Consequently, while agriculture may have increased the availability of food, it reduced the variety.

Types of Foods

The types of foods our ancestors ate can be described as **whole foods,** which suggests that our ancestors ate them pretty much as they came out of the ground, off the tree, or even off the hoof. In contrast, much of the food we eat today can be described as **partitioned foods,** foods from which some of the natural constituents have been removed. Partitioning is not necessarily bad. For example, whole milk contains fat that has been removed from skim milk, which many doctors prefer their patients with histories of heart disease to drink. However, many foods are reduced in quality when they are partitioned. For example, bleached flour, extracted from wheat seed, contains only starch, not the fiber and vitamins of whole-wheat flour. Many partitioned foods contain few nutrients. Other foods are **processed.** They have gone through a treatment, such as **refinement,** in which the coarse materials are removed, or **enrichment,** in which nutrient material is added.

Much of the processing and partitioning of food has been the result of improvement in processing machinery. For much of history, the processing of wheat to flour involved milling the entire seed, including the seed coat, the **bran;** the embryonic wheat plant, the **germ;** and the stored food for the young plant, the **endosperm.** The bran is a source of fiber, the germ a source of a variety of vitamins and minerals, and the endosperm a source of starch. The improvement of milling machinery initially eliminated the bran from flour and later the germ as well, reducing the nutrient value of the finished product. Because the more highly refined flour was whiter and apparently purer, it was incorrectly assumed to be of higher quality. It was the **Enrichment Act of 1942** that required that some nutrients be artificially reintroduced into refined flour and allowed the producers of products made from such flour to label their products **enriched,** while the more wholesome **whole-wheat products** could not be so labeled.

Nutrient Needs

The science of nutrition is concerned with the various chemicals within food that are referred to as **nutrients.** These are required for the health and maintenance of the human body. Inadequate consumption of a particular nutrient can lead to a **deficiency,** but defining what constitutes adequate consumption is difficult.

Minimum Daily Requirements (MDRs). Before requirements could be established, nutrients had to be identified. This effort began around 1880 when scientists first began to study deficiency diseases. During the 1950s, health scientists recommended that people consume their **Minimum Daily Requirements (MDRs)** for all nutrients. The MDRs were the smallest amounts a person needed to consume in order to avoid deficiencies. People were advised to eat minimum amounts because some nutrients are known to be toxic when taken in excess.

Recommended Dietary Allowances (RDAs). More recently, a committee of the **Food and Nutrition Board (FNB) of the National Academy of Sciences/National Research Council (NAS/NRC)** has been making **recommendations** concerning what people should be eating. (The government funds the FNB and appoints its members, who then function as independent scientists.) These **Recommended Dietary Allowances (RDAs)** (Table 1, pp. 8–9) for Americans, and the similar **Recommended Nutrient Intakes (RNIs)** for Canadians, have been established for vitamins, minerals, protein, and calories, and they change somewhat as new information becomes available. These recommendations consider that there are dissimilarities among people of different ages and sexes, unlike the MDRs, which were established for all people.

Diversity of need. All people do not need identical amounts of all nutrients. A given person's need for a specific nutrient may differ from someone else's, but all people fall within a definite **range** of needs; that is, there is a specific minimum and maximum between which all peoples' needs fall. In general, men are larger than women. Consequently, it would be reasonable that, again in general, men would have higher nutrient needs than women. Children, of course, are smaller than adults, but because they are growing, their needs for a specific nutrient may actually be higher than that of an adult. Biological events, such as pregnancy and lactation, and changes that occur with age, such as menopause, can also alter nutrient needs.

Consequently, the RDAs are set for specific *groups* of people. There are recommendations for infants; children up to age 10; males from age 11 through adulthood; nonpregnant, nonlactating females from age 11 through adulthood; pregnant females; and lactating females. Each group is further subdivided by age. For example, a male at 14 years of age has a higher vitamin D requirement than one over 25. But keep in mind that a random sample of ten 25-year-old men might show each with a different requirement for a given nutrient.

Actual individual requirements for some nutrients can be determined by a **balance study,** in which the difference between the amount of a nutrient consumed and that excreted, provided the nutrient is excreted without being altered, is measured. Such studies show a range in requirements, but if a large enough population of people is studied, they show that the needs of most individuals tend to cluster around a point near the middle of the range. If a large, random sample of individuals is tested, and the individuals' needs are plotted on a graph, the graph will resemble a bell (**bell-shaped curve**). See Figure 1. In a truly random population, the midpoint, or **median,** of the curve will be very, very close, if not identical, to the mathematical average, or **mean,** of the curve. The needs of half of the population would fall above the mean; the needs of the other half would fall below.

A BELL-SHAPED CURVE

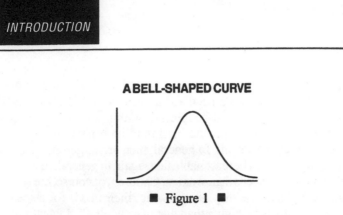

■ Figure 1 ■

In order to arrive at its recommendation, the FNB committee reviews studies that have been conducted and then sets its recommendation toward the largest nutrient requirement (Table 1). This way, the needs of most people are covered. It must be remembered that the committee makes recommendations that satisfy *most people's* needs; it does not set requirements that will satisfy everybody's. Furthermore, the recommendations set are to *maintain* health; disease conditions or any kind of fasting, including dieting and starvation, can increase one's needs.

There are three exceptions to the general RDA practice of listing highest nutrient requirements: **sodium, chlorine,** and **potassium.** Sodium and chlorine are found together in table salt, which has been linked to high blood pressure. Diets high in table salt can aggravate cases of high blood pressure and may lead to heart disease or stroke. A sodium recommendation that's safe for healthy people may worsen a bad condition in someone with high blood pressure. Consequently, a minimum recommendation is made for these two nutrients. Potassium is chemically related to sodium; *too little* potassium can be dangerous, although too much from food does not seem to be a problem. Therefore, a minimum recommendation is made also for potassium.

Energy RDA

Energy, measured in **calories,** is treated differently from the chemical nutrients. While an excess of most chemical nutrients is not harmful unless it is carried to an extreme, even a slight excess of calories over a period of time can lead to unwanted weight gain and even, eventually, to obesity. The committee determined average needs for people in its age/sex groups and set the calorie RDA at that level. Some latitude is built into those recommendations to accommodate larger or smaller individuals. Some foods may contain abundant calories but little other nutrition. Such foods, such as candy or other so-called "junk foods," may be described as sources of **empty calories,** that is, containing few nutrients per calorie. In contrast, foods such as fresh fruits, which provide vitamins, minerals, and fiber along with their calories, would be described as **nutrient-dense** foods. The energy RDA is best met from such foods. Otherwise, one may meet it but consume insufficient chemical nutrients.

Food Labels

The **Nutrition Education and Labeling Act of 1990** required that nutrition information on **food labels** conform to certain standards. For one thing, all ingredients of processed foods must be listed in order of decreasing quantity by weight. For example, hot cocoa mix usually contains more sugar than any other ingredient and consequently must list sugar first on its list of ingredients. Such information often requires some reader sophistication in order to interpret. That same product may list high-fructose corn syrup somewhere farther down on the list. Fructose is a type of sugar, and although it is not identical to table sugar, it is still a sweetener, and it still provides calories. In addition, the average person may not be acquainted with ingredients like sodium caseinate or cellulose gum or know what "partially hydrogenated" vegetable oil is.

    Among the "nutrition facts" given on food labels is a list of chemical nutrients in terms of their quantity and percentage of their respective RDAs. Since RDAs vary so much from group to group, providing an accurate label listing of RDA percentage is virtually impossible. Consequently, food producers use a separate standard called the **Reference Daily Intakes (RDIs)** (Table 1). RDIs cover the chemical nutrients, correspond to the RDAs, and are generally based on the

U.S. RECOMMENDED DIETARY ALLOWANCES (RDAs) FOR NUTRIENTS

Vitamins and Minerals

Age in years or circumstances	Weight (kg)	Weight (lb)	Height (cm)	Height (inches)	Protein (g)	Vitamin A (RE)	Vitamin D (µg)	Vitamin E (mg)	Vitamin K (µg)	Vitamin C (mg)	Thiamin (mg)	Riboflavin (mg)	Niacin (mg equiv.)	Vitamin B6 (mg)	Folate (µg)	Vitamin B12 (µg)	Calcium (mg)	Phosphorus (mg)	Magnesium (mg)	Iron (mg)	Zinc (mg)	Iodine (µg)	Selenium (µg)
Infants																							
0.0–0.5	6	13	60	24	13	375	7.5	3	5	30	0.3	0.4	5	0.3	25	0.3	400	300	40	6	5	40	10
0.5–1.0	9	20	71	28	14	375	10.0	4	10	35	0.4	0.5	6	0.6	35	0.5	600	500	60	10	5	50	15
Children																							
1–3	13	29	90	35	16	400	10.0	6	15	40	0.7	0.8	9	1.0	50	0.7	800	800	80	10	10	70	20
4–6	20	44	112	44	24	500	10.0	7	20	45	0.9	1.1	12	1.1	75	1.0	800	800	120	10	10	90	20
7–10	28	62	132	52	28	700	10.0	7	30	45	1.0	1.2	13	1.4	100	1.4	800	800	170	10	10	120	30
Males																							
11–14	45	99	157	62	45	1000	10.0	10	45	50	1.3	1.5	17	1.7	150	2.0	1200	1200	270	12	15	150	40
15–18	66	145	176	69	59	1000	10.0	10	65	60	1.5	1.8	20	2.0	200	2.0	1200	1200	400	12	15	150	50
19–24	72	160	177	70	58	1000	10.0	10	70	60	1.5	1.7	19	2.0	200	2.0	1200	1200	350	10	15	150	70
25–50	79	174	176	70	63	1000	5.0	10	80	60	1.5	1.7	19	2.0	200	2.0	800	800	350	10	15	150	70
51+	77	170	173	68	63	1000	5.0	10	80	60	1.2	1.4	15	2.0	200	2.0	800	800	350	10	15	150	70

Females

10–14	46	101	157	62	46	800	10.0	8	45	50	1.1	1.3	15	1.4	150	2.0	1200	1200	280	15	12	150	45
11–18	55	120	163	64	44	800	10.0	8	55	60	1.1	1.3	15	1.5	180	2.0	1200	1200	300	15	12	150	50
19–24	58	128	164	65	46	800	10.0	8	60	60	1.1	1.3	15	1.6	180	2.0	1200	1200	280	15	12	150	55
25–50	63	138	163	64	50	800	5.0	8	65	60	1.1	1.3	15	1.6	180	2.0	800	800	280	15	12	150	55
50+	65	143	160	63	50	800	5.0	8	65	60	1.0	1.2	13	1.6	180	2.0	800	800	280	10	12	150	55

Pregnant

	60					800	10.0	10	65	70	1.5	1.6	17	2.2	400	2.2	1200	1200	320	30	15	175	65

Lactating

First 6 months	65					1300	10.0	12	65	95	1.6	1.8	20	2.1	280	2.6	1200	1200	355	15	19	200	75
Second 6 months	62					1200	10.0	11	65	90	1.6	1.7	20	2.1	260	2.6	1200	1200	340	15	16	200	75

DAILY REFERENCE VALUES (DRVs)*

Food Component	DRV
fat	65 g
saturated fatty acids	20 g
cholesterol	300 mg
total carbohydrate	300 g
fiber	25 g
sodium	2400 mg
potassium	3500 mg
protein**	50 g

REFERENCE DAILY INTAKES (RDIs)

Nutrient	Amount	Nutrient	Amount
vitamin A	5000 IU	vitamin B_6	2.0 mg
vitamin C	60 mg	folic acid	0.4 mg
thiamin	1.5 mg	vitamin B_{12}	6 µg
riboflavin	1.7 mg	phosphorus	1.0 g
niacin	20 mg	iodine	150 µg
calcium	1.0 g	magnesium	400 mg
iron	18 mg	zinc	15 mg
vitamin D	400 IU	copper	2 mg
vitamin E	30 IU	biotin	0.3 mg
		pantothenic acid	10 mg

■ Table 1 ■

* Based on 2,000 calories a day. ** DRV for protein varies for certain populations; Reference Daily Intake (RDI) for protein has been established for children 1 to 4 years (16 g), infants under 1 year (14 g), pregnant women (60 g), nursing mothers (65 g).

high-end nutrient needs of adult males. But because women in their reproductive years have higher iron needs than do other age/sex groups because of menstruation, the RDI for iron corresponds to the needs of these women. In addition, nutrition facts labels also indicate **Daily Reference Values** (Table 1) for foods like fats and fiber, which are not covered by the RDAs.

Food Groups

Describing nutrient requirements in terms of chemistry may provide specific information for consumers, but by its nature, the information is not in practical terms. Few people read food information labels in order to gauge their nutrient intakes. But most people *are* acquainted with food types, so nutrition information has often been provided in terms of **food groups.** For many years, foods were separated into four basic groups: **grains, meats, dairy,** and **fruits and vegetables.** The names were pretty straightforward. **Grains** included not only whole grains, but also cereals, breads, pasta, and anything that was made from grains. **Dairy** was milk and anything that could be made from it, such as cheese, and it also included eggs. **Meats** covered virtually all nondairy animal products, including fish, shellfish, and poultry, as well as red meat. **Fruits and vegetables** included the foods that were derived from plants other than the grains. People were encouraged to eat from all four groups in order to achieve **a balanced diet.**

While the **basic four** food groups were easy to understand, they were not entirely accurate. Some foods, such as bacon or butter, were apparently members of the meat and dairy groups respectively, but they had little in common with the members of those groups nutritionally. Foods like corn and sometimes rice are eaten in the United States and Canada as vegetables, but technically, they are grains. Potatoes, while technically a vegetable and eaten that way, are nutritionally similar to many grains. And certain beans and nuts, again vegetables, are actually similar enough to meats to be substituted for them.

Another food classification system, the **basic seven,** included beans and nuts in the same group as meats, along with eggs. It also separated the fruits and vegetables into three groups: leafy green and yellow vegetables which are eaten cooked; citrus fruits, raw cabbage, tomatoes, and salad greens; and noncitrus fruits, potatoes, and other vegetables. It also separated butter and fortified margarine from the dairy group. This system identified specific nutrients provided by each group and recommended a specific number of daily servings from each of them.

The Food Guide Pyramid

More recently, the food group idea has been modified to six groups, and it is now presented in a way that is easy to understand and makes nutritional sense. In principle, the new scheme is similar to the basic four food groups, but vegetables and fruits are each in a category of its own. In addition, current wisdom has it that the grains should be the most heavily eaten of all categories: six to eleven servings per day. Vegetables should be consumed in the next greatest quantity: three to five servings per day. Fruits should be next: two to four servings per day. Dairy products and meats and meat substitutes should be eaten more sparingly. Two to three servings per day for each group is recommended. This plan can be represented in the shape of a **pyramid** (Figure 2). Grains make up the base of the pyramid; the vegetable and fruit groups are the next tier up. Meat and dairy groups compose the third tier. Finally, the apex of the pyramid is what might be called the fats, sweets, junk food, and dessert category. These foods should be consumed only sparingly. The food guide pyramid makes sense as long as one is eating whole foods, or at least nutrient-dense foods. Partitioned foods are often low in nutrients, and processing can add fat, salt, and sugar.

THE FOOD GUIDE PYRAMID

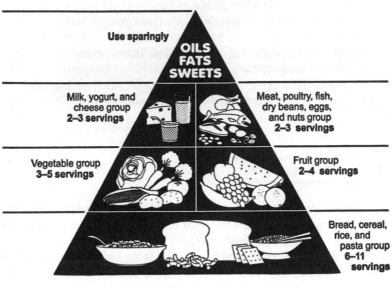

■ Figure 2 ■

Exchange Lists

People who follow a precise diet, such as diabetics or those trying to control their weight, may want something more exact than the food group plans. Such people are concerned with the quality of what they eat as well as the quantity; that is, they want to be well nourished, but they want to limit their intake. **Exchange lists** concentrate on serving size and nutrient content. In addition, they also consider the chemical nature of the food. Thus, cheese can be substituted, or exchanged, for meat because the two are similar in protein and fat content. Similarly, peas or potatoes, starchy vegetables, are comparable to grains. Foods like hot dogs, while popularly thought of as meat, are listed as fats, which, chemically, are more or less what many are. A person who uses exchange lists along with the food pyramid can easily obtain the appropriate RDAs for nutrients but at reduced calories.

Food Safety

Many students will recall an outbreak of food poisoning among children who had visited fast-food restaurants, part of a national chain in the Seattle, Washington, area in 1993. Many of the children became seriously ill; some died. The cause of the outbreak was determined to be meat contaminated with a type of bacteria called *E. coli* (technically *Escherichia coli*). The hamburgers made from the meat were not adequately cooked to kill the organisms. Such outbreaks have also occurred recently in the United States (from unpasteurized apple juice) and in Japan.

E. coli is a common inhabitant of the digestive systems of warm-blooded animals, including ourselves. Although it is generally harmless, there are dangerous strains such as the one that killed the children. There are a number of disease-causing organisms that are capable of being transmitted in contaminated food, typhoid fever and hepatitis among them. Other types of organisms may not cause disease *per se*, but if they grow in food and are eaten, their waste products may make us ill, as in the case of botulism, a poison often found in improperly canned foods.

In the past, food preservation was less than a precise science, and anyone purchasing food, say at an open market, was often taking chances. There was no way of knowing that food, particularly meat, bought in that manner was not spoiled. The government agency now charged with maintaining food safety is the **Food and Drug Administration (FDA)**. Food producers, processors, sellers, and servers are obligated to adhere to standards of hygiene and sanitation enforced by the FDA. Unfortunately, the FDA cannot be in all places at all times, and violations may occur.

Food preservation may be accomplished by a number of means. **Refrigeration** is one such method, which inhibits, or at least slows, the growth of organisms that can cause food spoilage. Milk undergoes **pasteurization,** a heating process that kills disease-causing organisms but essentially does not alter the milk. Canned foods must be **sterilized** as part of the canning process, killing not only the organisms on the food, but also the spores that could later germinate into new organisms. Canned foods are subjected to intense heat and pressure to accomplish sterilization, and the most frequent instances of poisoning involving canned foods occur with those canned improperly at home. Certain food **additives,** that is, chemicals deliberately added to foods, are used to prevent spoilage. In the past, sugar and salt were used toward this end, but more potent chemicals have replaced them. There have been questions raised about the safety of some of those additives for human consumption, and the FDA is responsible for ensuring it. Those additives that are used specifically to prevent spoilage are known as **preservatives** because their function is to preserve food freshness.

Special Diets

The term **diet** often connotes an eating plan that is reduced in calories with the specific goal of bringing about weight loss. In reality, a diet is simply what a person eats. Some diets may conform to cultural or ethnic guidelines; others may follow medical guidance. Some diets arise out of popular whim or misconception. Such **fad diets** generally promise weight loss, but others have offered energy, disease resistance or cure, or perhaps even more compelling, sexual prowess. Such diets often concentrate on a **gimmick,** a trick of some sort, as did the "grapefruit diet" of several years ago, which advocated eating grapefruit or drinking grapefruit juice with every meal. Its gimmick was that grapefruit somehow "burned" calories out of food. Grapefruit is a nourishing food, but it does not burn calories out of anything, and whenever a single food is stressed, it often pushes others out of the diet which may contain essential nutrients. Such fad diets can often lead to deficiencies.

BASIC CHEMISTRY

Matter and Energy

As an undergraduate years ago, I had a chemistry professor who took great delight in telling his students that if the human body could be broken down into its component chemicals and those chemicals packaged and sold, the total sale price would be under three dollars. Undoubtedly, inflation has done something to the price by now, but the professor's fundamental point is still valid: The human body is basically a collection of chemicals. In fact, all material in the universe, collectively referred to as **matter** and defined as anything that takes up space and has mass, is made up of chemicals. The remaining component of the universe is **energy**, which is defined as the ability to do work on matter, or make matter move. Energy is measured in **calories.** One calorie is the amount of energy needed to increase the temperature of a gram of water one degree Celsius. The familiar food calorie is actually a **kilocalorie,** 1000 calories, or the amount of energy needed to raise a kilogram of water one degree Celsius. For the remainder of this review, the term *calorie* will refer to the food calorie.

Elements and Compounds

Elements. If all of the naturally occurring matter in the universe could be collected and broken down into its basic components which were then divided into separate piles, there would be a total of 92 piles. These basic components of matter are the **elements,** or the simplest kinds of matter. There are actually more than 92 kinds of elements, but only 92 occur naturally. The remainder have been synthesized in laboratories. The smallest physical entity in which an element can exist is an **atom.** Atoms have been called the building blocks of elements, much as bricks are the building blocks of a brick wall.

Each atom (Figure 3) is itself made of smaller, or subatomic, particles, and atoms are distinguished from one another by the number of such particles they contain. The principal particles are the **proton,** which contains a positive electric charge, and an uncharged **neutron.** These are found together in the core, or **nucleus,** of the atom. A much smaller **electron,** which contains a negative charge that is equal and opposite that of the proton, orbits around the nucleus. Normally there are as many electrons in orbit as there are protons in the nucleus.

DIAGRAM OF AN ATOM

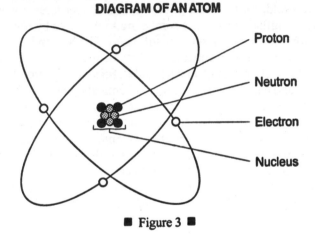

■ Figure 3 ■

Compounds. Elements can be combined to form new kinds of matter with properties that are different from those of the elements. For example, two gases, hydrogen and oxygen, can be combined in proper amounts to form the liquid water. Such combinations of elements are called **compounds.** When one is combining elements to form compounds, one is actually combining atoms to form **molecules.** The molecule is the building block of a compound just as the atom is the building block of an element.

Atoms combine, or **bond,** in two different ways. Under specified conditions, such as when dissolved in water, some atoms may lose or gain one or more electrons. An atom that has lost or gained an electron is an **ion.** Atoms gaining electrons become negatively charged anions, while those losing electrons become positively charged **cat-ions.** Anions and cations mutually attract each other, often strongly enough to bond together. Bonds formed between ions are called **ionic bonds.** Table salt is a compound that is formed by ionic bonding between cationic sodium and anionic chlorine. Other atoms do not physically give up electrons but may form bonds by sharing them with other atoms. In this case, each atom contributes an electron to be shared, and bonds formed in this manner are called **covalent bonds.** In the gas carbon dioxide, carbon and oxygen bond covalently. Atoms that form covalent bonds may share up to four pairs of electrons. Sometimes the sharing is unequal; that is, the shared electron pair is held more tightly by one atom than by the other. Bonds formed in this manner are intermediate between covalent and ionic bonding; they are called **polar covalent bonds.** Water is a compound formed by the polar covalent bonding of hydrogen and oxygen. The electrons are more tightly held by the oxygen than by hydrogen. Neither type of atom forms a true ion, but a molecule held together by a polar covalent bond may mimic one held together ionically in that there may be a positive and negative "pole" on the molecule.

Chemists divide compounds into two rough, major groups: **organic compounds** and **inorganic compounds.** Organic compounds contain the elements carbon and hydrogen specifically. Inorganic compounds may contain any combination of chemicals including carbon or hydrogen, but not both. Carbon atoms have a unique property of being capable of forming covalent bonds with other carbon atoms to the point where they may form long chains. This property allows for the formation of a vast number of organic compounds, perhaps as many as or more than all inorganic compounds. Usually carbon atoms share only a single pair of electrons between them; they form a **single covalent bond,** which can be represented as

$$-\overset{|}{\underset{|}{C}}-\overset{|}{\underset{|}{C}}-$$

Less frequently, a pair of carbon atoms may share two pairs of electrons to form a **double covalent bond,** which is represented as

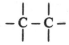

Rarely, a pair of carbon atoms may share three pairs of electrons and form a **triple covalent bond,** represented as

$$- C \equiv C -$$

Carbon atoms are capable of sharing four pairs of electrons, but never with another carbon atom. Quadruple bonds are unknown. An organic compound that contains only carbon and hydrogen is a **hydrocarbon.** A hydrocarbon that contains only single bonds along the carbon chain is a **saturated** hydrocarbon, and one with a double bond is **unsaturated.** If there are several points of unsaturation, the compound is **polyunsaturated** (Figure 4).

HYDROCARBONS

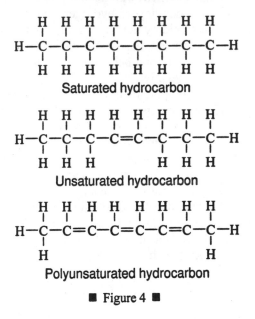

Saturated hydrocarbon

Unsaturated hydrocarbon

Polyunsaturated hydrocarbon

■ Figure 4 ■

Energy is often required in the formation of covalent bonds, and some of that energy may be released when those bonds are broken.

Chemical Nutrients

Just as the human body is a collection of chemicals, so is the food that nourishes it. Each nutrient has a specific role to play. Some nutrients provide energy, while others provide structural material. Others provide functional chemicals that assist in body processes, and still others act as regulators of body processes. There are six categories of **chemical nutrients,** each of which will be discussed in its own chapter. However, each is briefly introduced here.

Organic nutrients. Four of the nutrient categories, the **carbohydrates, lipids, proteins,** and **vitamins,** are organic compounds. Of these, all but vitamins are eaten in sufficient quantity to provide calories; consequently, they are often referred to as **energy nutrients.**

    Carbohydrates, described in the chapter beginning on page 53, contain the elements carbon, hydrogen, and oxygen roughly in a ratio of 2:1:1. Carbohydrates are generally used for quick bursts of energy, for example during a sprint. Certain organs of the body, specifically the brain and the nerves, use carbohydrates for their energy preferentially. There are two broad categories of carbohydrates: **simple carbohydrates,** or **sugars,** and **complex carbohydrates,** or **starches.** Sugars are naturally provided by fruits, some vegetables, and, to a lesser extent, milk. Sugar is added, often generously, to numerous processed foods, especially desserts, soft drinks, and candies, and many people use refined sugar in things they eat. Starches are found in grains, grain products such as pasta, grain substitutes, and some vegetables. Another group of complex carbohydrates is the indigestible **fiber,** which is normally found in whole grains, fruits, and vegetables. Even though fiber cannot be digested, it is still an important component of the diet. It helps maintain the health and proper functioning of the digestive system, particularly the large intestine.

    Lipids are usually divided into two subcategories: **fats** and **sterols.** Like the carbohydrates, lipids are composed of hydrogen, carbon, and oxygen, but oxygen is present in comparably minute amounts.

Fat on people generally represents stored energy, that is, calories that were eaten but not used. Regardless of the nutrient the excess calories came from, they are converted to and stored as **fat.** In the diet, fats are provided principally by animal foods, that is, meats and dairy products; however, certain grains and vegetables contain fats as well. Animal fats are typically saturated, which will be discussed in detail in the chapter on lipids (p. 69), and are solid. Lard, or pork fat, and tallow, or beef fat, are more or less familiar examples of saturated fats. In contrast, plant fats are typically unsaturated, are liquid in nature, and are generally referred to as **oils.** The fats, like the carbo-hydrates, are principally used for energy. Fats fuel low-intensity, en-durance types of activities such as walking, long-distance jogging, and aerobic dancing. **Sterols,** on the other hand, are not considered to be nutrients. Most sterols are not eaten; they are made internally, including perhaps the best known of them: **cholesterol.** Most people have heard about cholesterol, and they are aware of its relationship to heart disease. What is often not realized, however, is that most people make cholesterol in their livers from dietary saturated fat. It is usu-ally this cholesterol that plugs up their arteries, not the cholesterol they eat. Some amount of cholesterol in the blood is necessary for the transport of fats, which do not dissolve in blood as do other nutrients. In addition, a number of other biologically important chemicals are made from cholesterol. These include a number of hormones, includ-ing the reproductive hormones and the adrenal hormones. Again, all of this will be considered in detail later.

Food processing and preparation often add carbohydrates and fat, which add calories, to otherwise nourishing foods. For example, French-fried potatoes are prepared by immersion in boiling animal fat or oil, some of which is absorbed into the fries. In contrast, whole potatoes contain virtually no fat. In addition, many snack foods con-tain vast amounts of sugar (and calories) but little else. Foods that provide calories from fat or sugar but few or no other nutrients are popularly called **junk foods.** The energy they provide has been la-beled **empty calories.**

Proteins are unique among the energy nutrients in three ways. First, unlike carbohydrates and lipids, proteins contain the element nitrogen in addition to carbon, hydrogen, and oxygen. Second, the principal function of proteins is not to provide calories. Although protein is used for energy when carbohydrates are not sufficiently available, its main use is structural. Proteins are the primary chemical in most body tissues. In addition, the chief functional chemicals in the body, the **enzymes,** are also constructed from protein. The third way in which protein differs from the other energy nutrients is that it is a **macromolecule;** that is, proteins are very large molecules made of smaller molecular components, in this case **amino acids.** Most Americans rely on meat and dairy products for high-quality protein, but the majority of humans combine vegetable sources like nuts and beans with grain to adequately meet their protein needs.

The fourth of the organic nutrients is the **vitamins.** Unlike the others, there is no chemical consistency among the vitamins. Some contain nitrogen, and some do not. Some are soluble in water, and others are soluble in fat. Vitamins do not provide energy. They are consumed only in minute amounts, and some can be toxic if they are overconsumed. For the most part, they function as **regulators;** that is, they help in controlling a number of cell functions. Vitamins are described as **essential nutrients,** which means that they cannot be made internally but must be provided in the diet.

Inorganic nutrients. The remaining two categories of nutrients are the inorganic **minerals** and **water.**

Minerals are elements. Like the vitamins, they are essential nutrients. Some, also like the vitamins, function as regulators. Others are structural, and others still are essential participants in biological processes.

Water is technically not a nutrient. However, it is still an important part of the diet because, if for no other reason, it replaces the water that's lost every day through perspiration, urination, and respiration. Water makes up about 60% of the mass of the human body. Loss of too much of it, or **dehydration,** can lead to a number of bodily malfunctions, including death.

Alcohol

A potent source of calories but no other nutrients is **alcohol.** The idea of a "beer gut" is pretty well known, although it's likely that many of the calories responsible for the gut came from calories in snacks, like potato chips and pizza, as much as they did from the beer, although there is some carbohydrate in beer, a source of some of its calories. Distilled spirits contain fewer calories per serving, but they contain much more alcohol; consequently, their servings are smaller. Alcoholic drinks should not be considered a source of energy, however. The processing of the alcohol is accomplished by the liver, and long-term alcohol consumption can bring about the destruction of the liver through a disease called **cirrhosis.** Other organs, like the kidneys, can also be affected by long-term alcohol consumption. Furthermore, the short-term effects of alcohol on the digestive system and brain are well known. Alcohol consumption, when coupled with driving, is responsible for many thousands of traffic fatalities every year. The biological and social consequences of alcohol make it a lousy source of energy.

People, like all other animals, are composed of trillions of microscopic units known as **cells.** Each cell is capable of carrying on most, if not all, of the characteristics of life, including respiration, metabolism, and in some cases reproduction.

Cell Structure

Each cell is composed of smaller structures called **organelles** (Figure 5). The word means exactly what it looks like: small organs. By analogy, the organelles have a similar relationship to our cells that organs have to our bodies.

The outer covering of animal cells is an envelope made of lipid and protein that is known as the **plasma membrane** or **cell membrane.** It is described as being **semipermeable** (although **selectively permeable** is probably a better description), which means that it is capable of allowing some materials to penetrate and enter the cell while it keeps others out.

Movement through the Plasma Membrane

Some material is capable of moving through the cell membrane by simple **diffusion.** If there is a greater concentration of the material outside the cell than inside, that is, if there is a **concentration gradient** toward the inside of the cell, the material flows in until it is equally concentrated on both sides of the membrane. This is similar to smoke spreading through an open door from a room where someone is smoking to a room where no one is.

THE COMPONENTS OF A CELL

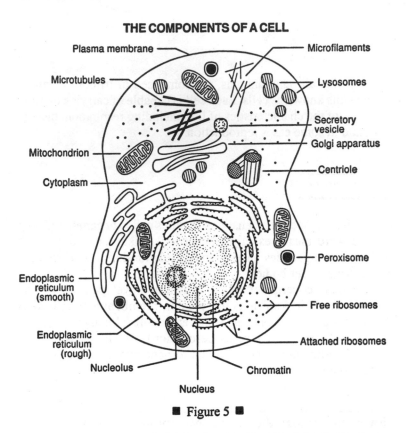

Plasma membrane — Microfilaments

Microtubules — Lysosomes

Secretory vesicle

Golgi apparatus

Mitochondrion — Centriole

Cytoplasm

Peroxisome

Endoplasmic reticulum (smooth)

Free ribosomes

Endoplasmic reticulum (rough)

Attached ribosomes

Nucleolus — Chromatin

Nucleus

■ Figure 5 ■

Water passes through a cell membrane by the process of **osmosis**. In this case, water follows an inverse salt gradient, which can be demonstrated by putting a raw French fry in a glass of salty water. The salt draws water out of the cells of the piece of potato, making it limp. A similar phenomenon occurs if one eats a bag of salty potato chips without drinking anything. Salt draws water out of cells lining the mouth, giving the illusion of dryness and causing thirst.

Some materials may enter a cell only with an expenditure of energy, that is, by a cell working to absorb the material. This phenomenon is called **active transport**, and it involves the protein in the cell membrane, which may act as the entryway for the material. The energy for this process is provided by the chemical **adenosine triphosphate (ATP)**. When energy nutrients are broken down in the cell, ATP is formed as a temporary reservoir of energy. Cellular activities, such as contraction of a muscle cell or absorption of a molecule by active transport, use ATP for their fuel.

The Nucleus

The biggest organelle in the cell is usually the **nucleus,** where the hereditary information, or genes, is found. Genes are composed of **deoxyribose nucleic acid,** more commonly referred to as **DNA.** The information in the genes is expressed through the construction of specific proteins, many of which are enzymes—lactase, for example. A person who is unable to digest the sugar in milk lacks the enzyme to do it, lactase. His or her genes do not dictate the synthesis of the protein the enzyme is made of.

Cytoplasm, Mitochondria, and the Ultimate Breakdown of Food

Between the cell membrane and the nucleus is the gelatinous **cytoplasm,** within which the remaining organelles are found. Among them are the **mitochondria** (singular, **mitochondrion**)—the "powerhouses" of the cell. It is within the mitochondria that the products of food digestion are ultimately broken down and energy is released and temporarily held in the chemical **adenosine triphosphate (ATP).**

Breakdown usually begins in the cytoplasm, but it is not completed there. The remaining nutrient fragments are transported into the mitochondria, where the breakdown processes continue. Carbon and oxygen from the nutrients are removed together as **carbon dioxide** (CO_2), which is eliminated by the respiratory system. Hydrogen remains within the mitochondria and is ultimately combined with respiratory oxygen to form water (H_2O) that is removed by the kidneys. It is during the passage of hydrogen to oxygen that most ATP is formed. The oxygen needed for hydrogen removal is provided, of course, by breathing, the same method by which carbon dioxide is removed.

Much of the water that's formed is removed by urination, as indicated above, but some is lost across the skin by perspiration, and some is lost by breathing as well. Some, perhaps, may also be employed to provide the water the cells and tissues need to maintain themselves. (Some animals, such as the kangaroo rat of the American desert, do not drink but rather get their water from what they eat.)

Ribosomes and Protein Synthesis

Not all organelles are involved in the breakdown of chemicals. Some construct them. Among these are the **ribosomes,** which synthesize protein from amino acids. A chemical message from the nuclear DNA to the ribosomes dictates the structure the protein will take. Proteins synthesized by free-floating ribosomes in the cytoplasm are used within the cell. Some ribosomes that are embedded in a series of membranes known as the **endoplasmic reticulum** produce proteins that are exported from the cell as would be the case with digestive enzymes produced by cells lining the stomach, for example. Before a protein is exported from a cell, it is first packaged by another series of membranes, the **Golgi body,** or **Golgi apparatus.** The packaging material, actually a piece of the Golgi membrane, fuses with the plasma membrane on contact with it, dumping the protein contents outside the cell. **Secretory cells,** those that routinely produce proteins for export, have a very well-developed endoplasmic reticulum and Golgi apparatus.

Phagocytosis and Pinocytosis

The amino acids needed for protein synthesis are absorbed by the cells from the environment that surrounds them. Our own cells, like those of all animals, use dietary protein as the amino acid source. Cells normally absorb chemicals by the processes described above. Certain cells, however, occasionally engulf a small particle or bit of liquid by the processes of **phagocytosis** and **pinocytosis,** respectively. **Leukocytes,** or **white blood cells,** regularly carry on phagocytosis. They circulate through the blood toward sites of infection, where they engulf and digest the infecting organisms. Once the cell has ingested the infecting organism, it contains it in a cavity, the **vacuole,** into which another organelle, the **lysosome,** pours digestive enzymes.

Because cells are so small, they are able to get everything they need from the environment that surrounds them. In a large animal, such as a human, it is up to the organ systems to deliver those materials to the cells or, more appropriately, to their immediate environments. In the following chapters, these systems are described.

The Digestive Process

In order for the chemicals in our food to be made available to our cells and tissues, they must first undergo **digestion;** that is, they must be broken down to their chemical components, a process accomplished in two ways. First, the physical breakdown of food, including chopping, tearing, and grinding by our teeth as well as pulverization in the stomach and intestines, constitutes **mechanical digestion.** Second, the chemical breakdown of food by enzymes is called **chemical digestion.** Both processes take food at its bulk level and reduce it to its **molecular level,** that is, to the level of its component molecules. Once this breakdown has occurred, digested food can be **absorbed** into the circulatory system for transport to the various parts of the body. The digestive system consists of two basic components: the **alimentary canal,** or food tube, that runs from the mouth to the anus and the **associated organs** that provide digestive chemicals.

The Alimentary Canal

The mouth and teeth. Our bodies, like those of other complex organisms, can be described as a tube within a tube. The inner tube is the **alimentary canal.** It begins with the **mouth** and its organs of mechanical digestion: the **teeth.** Adults typically have 32 teeth divided into two sets of 16. One set occurs in the upper jaw, the **maxilla,** and one set occurs in the lower jaw, the **mandible.** Each set can be divided into symmetrical halves (Figure 6). The first two teeth in each half are the front teeth, or **incisors,** which are used for cutting. Going from front to rear, next to the incisors is a single **canine,** sometimes called the **fang,** particularly in animals in which it's well developed, such as cats and vampires. The canine is typically used for tearing. Next are the two **bicuspids (premolars).** The first of these

THE TEETH OF THE UPPER JAW

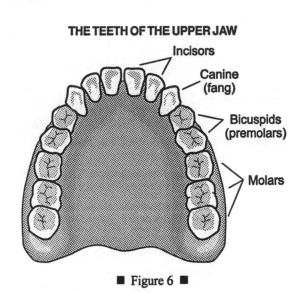

Incisors

Canine
(fang)

Bicuspids
(premolars)

Molars

■ Figure 6 ■

has a cutting edge toward the outside and is used to some degree for tearing, but toward the center, it is flat and, with the second bicuspid, is also used for grinding. Finally, there are three **molars,** flat-surfaced teeth that are used for grinding. The third molars are sometimes called the **wisdom teeth,** and they characteristically cause problems in many people whose jaws are simply not large enough to accommodate them.

Each tooth is divided into regions. The part extending out of the gums is the **crown.** The internal part, the **root,** is anchored firmly in the bone of the jaw. Between the two is a short **neck.** Teeth are somewhat similar to bone in composition, but their covering, the **enamel,** is the hardest substance in the human body. Immediately inside the enamel is the **dentin,** which is composed of a material similar to ivory. It extends through the root. Innermost in the tooth is the **pulp cavity,** which contains the nerve and a small blood vessel (Figure 7). Most of us are born without erupted teeth. The first teeth to develop

CROSS SECTION OF A PERMANENT TOOTH

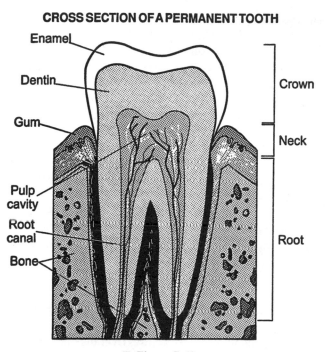

■ Figure 7 ■

are temporary, or **deciduous.** Often called milk teeth or baby teeth, they are lost during childhood and replaced by **permanent teeth.**

Also within the mouth is the **tongue.** It is covered with tiny projections, or **papillae** (singular, **papilla**), which are more commonly called the **taste buds.** Chemicals in solution excite nerve endings in the taste buds, which respond by sending a signal to the brain. This signal is interpreted as taste. There are only four basic flavors a human can taste—sweet, salt, sour, and bitter—and receptors for each have specific locations on the tongue. These are at the very tip (sweet), along the side toward the front (salt), along the side toward the rear (sour), and at the very rear (bitter). The chemicals initiating sweet and salt flavors are obvious enough. Sour is actually a sensation in response to acids, and bitter is a response to something like quinine, the chemical that gives tonic water its characteristic flavor. These tastes have survival value. Naturally sweet foods, like fruits, are generally nutrient dense and nourishing. Our bodies generally need salt (which often was not readily available to our ancestors); consequently, salty foods appeal to us naturally. (People who are exposed to salt early in life often grow up craving it.) In contrast, bitter and sour materials may be poisonous. A natural reaction to such tastes is often to spit the material out. The rest of what is recognized as taste is actually smell that is caused as chemicals released from food in the mouth drift into the nasal cavities.

While the principal function of the teeth is the mechanical breakdown of food, the act of chewing also releases chemicals that are tasted and mixes food with secretions from the **salivary glands,** which will be described shortly.

The throat and esophagus. The **throat,** or more correctly the **pharynx,** begins at the back of the mouth and is where swallowing begins. During swallowing the **epiglottis** closes over the opening to the windpipe, preventing food from entering the respiratory system. Swallowing is a voluntary act, but once it has begun, everything that follows is involuntary. Swallowing pushes chewed food, now called a **bolus,** through the throat and into the **esophagus,** the tube that runs from the pharynx into the stomach. The esophagus is composed of **smooth,** or **involuntary, muscle** which functions without conscious control. Swallowing is followed by a wave of contraction of the esophageal muscle, **peristalsis,** that works from the top of the esophagus toward the bottom pushing the bolus toward the stomach. Where the esophagus joins the stomach, a ring of muscle, the **cardiac sphincter,** opens to allow the bolus to pass through. Normally, the sphincter is closed to keep the stomach contents from splashing up into the esophagus, where they could cause damage.

The stomach. The **stomach** is a muscular pouch, perhaps one to two liters in capacity. Food arriving at the stomach is subjected to more peristaltic activity as the stomach contracts. This activity serves to further break down food mechanically, but it also mixes the swallowed food with **gastric juice,** a secretion of cells embedded in the stomach lining. Gastric juice consists principally of **hydrochloric acid** and the enzyme **pepsin,** which works specifically on protein, partially digesting it. The peristaltic movement of the stomach also pushes food on toward the **pyloric sphincter,** the ring of muscle that separates the stomach from the small intestine. Food is passed through the pyloric sphincter bit by bit. (See Figure 8 for an illustration of the human digestive system.)

The small intestine. The **small intestine** is a serpentine tube, perhaps 20 feet in length, where the bulk of digestion and most **absorption** actually takes place. The initial section is the short **duodenum,** into which acidic, partially digested food, called **chyme,** is discharged from the stomach. Here, tubes from the **gallbladder** and **pancreas** (described shortly) carry **liver bile** and **pancreatic juice** into the duodenum. Both of these secretions are alkaline and neutralize the acidic chyme.

In addition, bile **emulsifies** any fat that's present. In order for enzymatic digestion to occur, food material must be suspended in water. Fat does not mix with water, but during **emulsification,** fat is broken down into microscopic droplets which are suspendable and which **lipase,** the fat-digesting enzyme in pancreatic juice, can handle. Pancreatic juice also contains protein and sugar-digesting enzymes.

The first ten feet or so of the intestine following the duodenum is **the jejunum;** the remainder is the **ileum.** Cells in the wall of the intestine secrete **intestinal juice,** a mixture of enzymes that finish the chemical digestion of food.

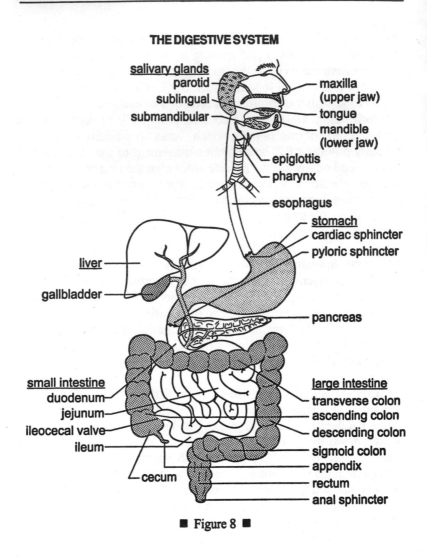

THE DIGESTIVE SYSTEM

salivary glands
   parotid
   sublingual
   submandibular

maxilla (upper jaw)
tongue
mandible (lower jaw)
epiglottis
pharynx
esophagus

stomach
cardiac sphincter
pyloric sphincter

liver
gallbladder
pancreas

small intestine
   duodenum
   jejunum
   ileocecal valve
   ileum
   cecum

large intestine
transverse colon
ascending colon
descending colon
sigmoid colon
appendix
rectum
anal sphincter

■ Figure 8 ■

The inner surface of the small intestine is covered with tiny projections called **villi** (singular, **villus**), which give it a velvety texture and appearance (Figure 9). Within these villi are microscopic blood vessels, **capillaries,** and a **lacteal, a lymph capillary** (see the following chapter). Molecules of food are absorbed into the villi and into the capillaries with the exception of digested fat, which enters the lacteal. The blood transports food molecules to the liver for further processing, and the digested fats are carried by the **lymphatic vessels** to eventually be deposited into the circulating blood in the vein coming up from the left arm. Whatever has not been digested and a large amount of water is transported by peristalsis to the end of the ileum where it passes through the **ileocecal valve,** a sphincter that separates the ileum from the large intestine.

SECTION THROUGH A VILLUS

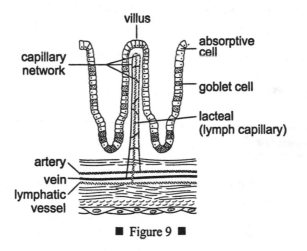

■ Figure 9 ■

The large intestine. The final part of the alimentary canal, the **large intestine,** or **colon,** is divided into four parts: the **ascending colon,** the **transverse colon,** the **descending colon,** and finally the **sigmoid colon.** Each of the first three is up to two feet in length. At the very beginning of the ascending colon, below the ileocecal valve, is a short section called the **cecum,** from which the **appendix** hangs.

The large intestine is the final processing point in the digestive system. No digestive enzymes are secreted here. Instead, undigested residues are attacked by **bacteria,** microscopic organisms that live within the large intestine. These break down many materials that we cannot and, in so doing, process them so that they can be eliminated. In the process, the bacteria secrete certain vitamins, particularly **vitamin K,** which we absorb and use. When certain materials, notably plant fibers and some sugars, are broken down, they undergo a gas-releasing process called **fermentation,** which accounts for the characteristic side effects of foods like baked beans. As residues are broken down, water is absorbed from them, and they are passed toward the very end of the large intestine, through the **sigmoid colon,** the short, curved section at the end, and into the **rectum,** a muscular pouch. A pair of **anal sphincters** separates the rectum from the outside. It is through these sphincters the final residue, now called **feces,** passes.

The Associated Organs

The salivary glands. There are three pairs of major **salivary glands** located around the mouth. The **sublingual glands** are under the tongue, the large **submandibular glands** are just inside the angle of the lower jaw, and the **parotid glands** are just in front of the ears. Salivary glands secrete **saliva** into the mouth through ducts. Saliva is mostly watery, but a thicker material, **mucus,** is also secreted, lubricating chewed food and making it easier to swallow. Saliva also contains an enzyme, **amylase,** which begins breaking starch down into sugar. Secretion of saliva is often in response to signals that trigger thoughts of food, such as cooking odors; however, chewing will start saliva flowing.

The liver. The **liver** performs several important functions in digestion, among which is the production and secretion of **bile.** Bile neither is an enzyme nor does it contain enzymes. Its function is like that of a detergent; it **emulsifies** fat; that is, it breaks it into tiny droplets that can be suspended in water and attacked by fat-digesting enzymes. Bile is secreted constantly, but it is stored in the **gallbladder,** a bulblike structure on the liver. The presence of fat in the upper small intestine triggers the release of a **hormone,** a regulatory chemical, from the intestine's inner surface. The hormone travels to the gallbladder by way of the blood and stimulates the gallbladder to contract and send bile down the **bile duct** into the duodenum.

The liver also has many roles to perform on digested food. Once food is absorbed into the blood capillaries in the villi, it is transported into larger and larger vessels, which finally collect into the **hepatic portal vein.** This vein carries nutrients from the small intestine to the liver, where some nutrients, specifically sugar and some vitamins and minerals, are stored until needed. In addition, the liver may convert some nutrients to others, such as excess proteins to sugar, if it's needed. Finally, food may contain some toxic materials. The liver converts many of these into nontoxic chemicals, with perhaps alcohol as the best example. Some compounds may defy conversion and may end up being stored by the liver instead.

The pancreas. The other major accessory organ of digestion is the **pancreas,** which lies behind the stomach. This organ produces and secretes a number of enzymes which are passed into the duodenum through the **pancreatic duct.** The same hormone that affects the gallbladder stimulates the pancreas to release **pancreatic juice.**

Digestive Disorders

There are many malfunctions that can occur within the digestive system. This review will consider only a few of the more common ones.

Dental caries. The most common digestive disorder is **dental caries,** better known as tooth decay, which results from bacterial breakdown of food debris on the teeth. The bacteria produce acidic waste products that erode the enamel and eat through the dentin, allowing the softer materials underneath to be invaded by bacteria. If the resulting infection gets deep into the roots, a puss-filled sac, or **abscess,** can form. This condition can be very painful, especially if the abscess is allowed to grow. Tooth decay is prevented, of course, by proper dental care.

Ulcers. Ulcers are irritated spots in either the stomach or duodenum that cause episodes of pain. The exact cause of these is not known, but they have been associated with nervous stress. However, most stomach, or **gastric,** ulcers are complicated by, and perhaps result from, bacterial infection. Such ulcers are more successfully treated with antibiotics than they are with traditional antacids and acid-blocking medications.

Gastritis. Gastritis is an irritation of the stomach lining. It may be caused by a viral infection, but it most usually results from some kind of abuse, for example, eating too much of the wrong thing, drinking too much, or even smoking too much.

Diverticulitis. This disease involves the development of small, sac-like swellings (**diverticula**) in the walls of the large intestine toward the anal end. This condition is called **diverticulosis.** If the diverticula become inflamed, the result is the painful condition **diverticulitis,** which, if left untreated, can lead to the formation of abscesses which, in turn, may perforate the large intestinal wall and lead to infections within the body cavity. Diverticulitis may result from a diet that is too low in fiber. Pushing on fiber strengthens the intestinal wall, while the absence of dietary fiber allows it to weaken and form diverticula. Diverticulitis rarely develops in Africa and Asia, where the diets are rich in fiber.

Hepatitis. Hepatitis is an inflammation of the liver. There are at least four types, three of which are caused by viruses. Viral infection may come about by a number of means, including ingesting the hepatitis virus, which can occur when someone eats or drinks something that has somehow been contaminated with fecal material of a carrier, for example, by drinking improperly treated, sewage-polluted water. Other means of infection include improperly treated acupuncture needles, tattooing, intravenous drug apparatus, blood transfusions, and even unprotected sex with an infected partner. The disease is characterized by **jaundice,** a yellowing of the skin and whites of the eyes, and it may include discoloration of urine, whitening of feces, abdominal discomfort, weakness, and nausea. Some forms can lead to death.

Gallbladder disease. More commonly known as **gallstones,** this disease involves the formation of crystals in the gallbladder. If a crystal lodges in and blocks the bile duct, the result is excruciating pain. The risk of gallbladder disease increases with age and overweight, and for some reason, women are more frequently afflicted than men. Sometimes, surgical removal of the gallbladder is the only cure for gallstones.

Cancer. Any part of the digestive system can develop **cancer,** and cancer in the large intestine is ranked third (below only lung cancer and breast cancer) in frequency in the United States. The cause of digestive cancers is not well known, but links with certain types of diets have been suggested. For example, people who eat a lot of smoked foods may be more at risk for stomach cancer, while those who eat little fiber may be more at risk for cancer in the large intestine. Whatever the cause may be, a nutritious and sensibly varied diet seems to be the best prevention.

The digestive system has the job of breaking down food to its molecular components and absorbing them. From that point, other organ systems distribute the digested food, provide other chemicals needed for using it, and remove any waste products that may be produced. Still other organ systems use the nutrients to carry out their services to the body, including the systems involved in processing food. Nutrients necessary to specific organ systems will be discussed later. A quick summary of the body's organ systems and how they affect or are affected by nutrition is provided here.

The Circulatory System

The **circulatory system** consists of the **blood,** the pump that makes it circulate—the **heart**—and the vessels through which the blood flows. The system is closed; the only way anything can normally enter and leave it is by diffusing through the vessel walls, and that can occur only through certain ones.

Blood. Blood consists of two principal components: the blood cells and the plasma. **Red blood cells** carry oxygen to the tissues, which the tissues use for extracting energy from nutrients. The less abundant but more varied **white blood cells** are involved in protection against disease. The **plasma,** the fluid component of the blood, is mostly water, but it also contains a number of **plasma proteins** such as **antibodies,** chemicals that function with the white blood cells. Other proteins are responsible for maintaining proper blood fluid concentration and bringing about clotting, when it's needed. In addition, the plasma contains materials being transported by the blood, such as hormones, nutrients, and waste materials.

The heart. The **heart** is a muscular organ that consists of four chambers: two **atria** (singular, **atrium**), which receive blood, and two **ventricles,** which pump it. The right atrium of the heart receives **deoxygenated blood,** blood that is returning from the tissues with no oxygen in the cells but carbon dioxide in the plasma. The right ventricle pumps the blood to the lungs, where the carbon dioxide is removed and oxygen is absorbed. The left atrium of the heart receives the **oxygenated blood** that returns from the lungs, and the left ventricle pumps it to the tissues. Each beat of the heart represents a pumping cycle. Heart rate is determined by a number of factors, including the demand for oxygen by the tissues.

The blood vessels. The **arteries** carry blood away from the heart. They are relatively thick walled and elastic in order to take the punishment of the rush of blood, or **pulse,** caused by each heartbeat. The **veins** carry blood to the heart. Their walls are less thick and elastic, and they contain periodic **valves,** particularly in the legs, to prevent backflow. Arteries branch into progressively smaller vessels as they get farther from the heart, and veins get progressively larger as they converge on their way toward the heart. Arteries and veins connect with each other at their smallest and most distant points from the heart through microscopic vessels called **capillaries.** Capillary beds service every part of the body. Capillary walls are just one cell thick, and through them material can be exchanged between the blood and tissues. Oxygen and nutrients diffuse from the blood into the tissues, and carbon dioxide and wastes diffuse from the tissues into the blood.

In the digestive system, nutrients diffuse into the capillaries of the villi. These capillaries converge into the **hepatic portal vein,** which flows not toward the heart but toward the liver. There the vessel branches again into capillaries so that digested nutrients can be absorbed into the liver, where some are stored and others are processed before they enter free circulation.

The Lymphatic System

The **lymphatic system** can be thought of as a secondary circulatory system. However, it is an open system. It's component fluid, **lymph,** is much like blood plasma; however, it contains fewer plasma proteins. Lymph is formed from fluid that diffuses from the blood through the capillaries and slowly flows through the tissues. It drains into the **lymph capillaries** which converge to form **lymph vessels.** Lymph is finally returned to the blood by way of **lymph ducts.** Lymph carries digested fat from the digestive system to the blood through the lymphatic system. There is no driving pump like the heart in the lymphatic system. Lymph is simply pushed along by hydrostatic pressure. But lymph vessels, like veins, have periodic valves to prevent backflow.

The lymphatic system is also a part of the **immune system,** which is specifically concerned with disease resistance. The immune system is not an easily defined, self-contained system such as the digestive system or circulatory system. It involves components of a number of other systems. At the points where lymphatic vessels converge are **lymph nodes,** glands in which white blood cells called lymphocytes, which are involved in disease resistance, or **immunity,** remain until they're needed. Lymph nodes often swell during an infection indicating that they are involved in the immune reaction.

Other lymphatic organs include the **tonsils,** the **spleen,** and the **thymus gland.** The **tonsils** are actually groups of lymph nodes. They are located at the back of the throat, where they help protect against oral and nasal bacteria that could become harmful. The tonsils often become inflamed in children. The **spleen** is the largest of the lymphatic organs. It is located toward the left end of the pancreas. It serves as a reservoir for red blood cells and detects the presence of foreign materials, such as disease organisms, in the blood. The **thymus gland** in a newborn baby is a large organ extending from the throat to the region of the heart, but in an adult only a remnant remains near the top of the heart. Early in life, the thymus is involved in the development of specific white blood cells called **T lymphocytes.** Some of these cells attack infective organisms, and others attack tumors. Other T lymphocytes act as regulators of immune response, and it is these cells that the AIDS virus appears to infect.

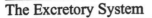

The Excretory System

The breakdown of nutrients in cells is an **oxidative** process; that is, it involves a reaction between oxygen and the nutrient, analogous to a fire, which is a reaction between oxygen and some kind of fuel. Also, as fire produces waste materials such as smoke and ash, the breakdown of nutrients also produces waste materials. The lungs, skin, gastrointestinal tract, and the urinary system all contribute to the elimination of waste from the body and constitute the **excretory system.**

The major organs of the **urinary system** (Figure 10) are the **kidneys.** The urinary system removes some of the body's waste materials, particularly **urea** from protein breakdown. Blood flows into the kidneys by way of a large artery which then branches into capillaries inside the kidney. From the capillaries, most of the blood's contents pass into the filtering units of the kidney, the **nephrons.** As the filtrate passes through the twisted tubing of the nephrons, capillaries running parallel to them absorb most of the filtrate back into the blood. The fluid that remains contains about a hundredth of the water that passed into it initially, some salts, and all of the urea. This mixture is urine. It passes from the nephrons into **collecting tubes,** which finally collect into a **ureter,** which carries the urine from the kidney to the **urinary bladder.** As the bladder accumulates urine, it stretches until it reaches its capacity. Release of urine through the **urethra** is a voluntary act. Frequency of urination is most affected by the amount of water one drinks; however, certain compounds, such as caffeine, stimulate urine formation. Such compounds are called **diuretics.**

THE URINARY SYSTEM

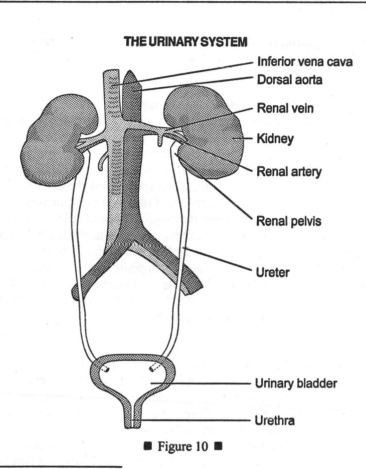

- Inferior vena cava
- Dorsal aorta
- Renal vein
- Kidney
- Renal artery
- Renal pelvis
- Ureter
- Urinary bladder
- Urethra

■ Figure 10 ■

The Nervous System

Nerves and nerve tissue. **Nerves** are composed of cells called **neurons,** which are specialized for conducting impulses. The neurons can pass an impulse to another neuron or to an organ or muscle. Nerve transmission coordinates the activities of the parts of the body, including some of the functioning of the digestive system.

The nervous system is divided into the **central nervous system,** which consists of the **brain** and **spinal cord,** and the **peripheral**

nervous system, which is made up of the remaining nervous tissue in the body.

The central nervous system. The human brain (Figure 11) receives **sensory** input from the peripheral nervous system and sends out **motor** impulses. Sensory input, from the mouth and nose, for example, is transmitted to the **cortex,** the outermost part of the brain and the location of consciousness and awareness. Beneath the cortex, immediately behind the bridge of the nose and toward the center of the head, is the **hypothalamus,** a region of the brain that monitors much of the general state of the body. It recognizes when nutrient and water concentrations in the blood become depleted, and it signals the cortex, which interprets the signals as hunger or thirst. The hypothalamus has also been called the center for appetite control. At the base of the brain, just above the spinal cord, is the **medulla oblongata,** which responds to odors, tastes, and even thoughts of food by sending impulses through a peripheral nerve to the stomach.

The peripheral nervous system. The **peripheral nerves** carry impulses to and from the brain and spinal cord. **Sensory nerves** typically carry information toward the central nervous system, and **motor nerves** carry them away from the central nervous system. Some motor nerves control voluntary activities, and some control involuntary activities, like digestion. Swallowing is the final voluntary act in digestion; the rest is involuntary and is controlled by the tenth cranial nerve, the **vagus nerve,** which carries impulses to the stomach and intestine from the medulla oblongata. (Cranial nerves are peripheral nerves that connect directly to the brain; they do not lead into the spinal cord.) The vagus affects a number of the body's functions that occur simultaneously with digestion. As digestion gets underway, particularly after a heavy meal, blood pressure typically falls, the heart slows, breathing becomes shallow, and one typically feels fatigued. As the vagus fires to affect digestion, it also brings about those other responses.

THE HUMAN BRAIN IN CROSS SECTION

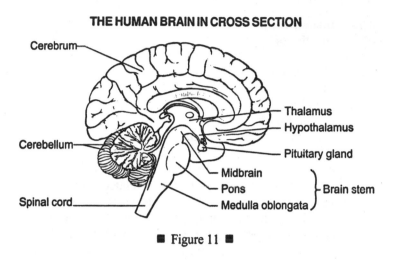

■ Figure 11 ■

The Endocrine System

The **endocrine system** is a collection of organs that produce regulatory chemicals called **hormones.** These hormones are released directly into the blood and do not pass through a duct or tube. Some endocrine glands have functions in addition to producing hormones, and some are involved directly or indirectly with the digestive system.

A gland closely associated with the hypothalamus is the **pituitary gland** (Figure 11). At one time, it was called the master gland because it secretes **tropic hormones,** which control other endocrine glands. One gland affected by the pituitary is the **thyroid gland** (Figure 12), which produces **thyroxine,** a hormone that controls the speed of **metabolism;** that is, it controls the rate at which the body functions. Some people tend to "burn" faster than others; that is, they tend to produce more thyroxine, have a high rate of metabolism, and may have a harder time keeping weight on. In contrast, people with a slower rate of metabolism produce less thyroxine. Such people may have a hard time losing weight, which is not to say that all weight-related problems involve a malfunction of the thyroid gland. Most don't. But the thyroid gland can be a factor in some cases. Production of thyroxine requires dietary iodine. If a diet lacks iodine, the thyroid gland swells in response, a condition called **goiter.** People with goiter are often heavy.

Immediately behind the thyroid gland are the **parathyroid glands** (Figure 12). The parathyroids are not controlled by tropic hormones; rather, the parathyroid hormone, **parathormone,** is secreted in response to calcium levels in the blood. Parathormone is responsible for inducing the intestine to absorb calcium for transfer into the blood.

Perhaps the best known of the nutrition-related endocrine glands is the **pancreas** (Figure 8, p. 34), the same organ that produces digestive enzymes. The endocrine parts of the pancreas are called the **islets of Langerhans.** They produce the hormones **insulin** and **glucagon,** hormones responsible for regulating blood sugar level. Insulin stimulates the liver and muscles to take up sugar when it is at a high level in the blood, such as after a meal heavy in carbohydrates. In contrast, glucagon stimulates the liver to release sugar back into the blood when the level is low, such as during a fast.

Other hormones function within the digestive system itself. **Gastrin,** secreted by the stomach and duodenum, increases the secretion of gastric juice, and it increases the movement of chyme out of the stomach by relaxing the pyloric sphincter. Nervous impulses from the medulla oblongata, by way of the vagus nerve, stimulate the release of gastrin, as does the presence of food, alcohol, or caffeine in the stomach. **Secretin** is secreted by the duodenum in response to the presence of acid chyme. This hormone inhibits the secretion of gastric juice and initiates the secretion of pancreatic juice, particularly that component that contains a chemical to neutralize the acid chyme. In addition, it promotes bile secretion. **Cholecystokinin,** secreted by the small intestine, promotes the secretion of pancreatic juice that is rich in digestive enzymes, and it stimulates the gallbladder to contract and eject bile into the duodenum.

THE THYROID AND PARATHYROID GLANDS

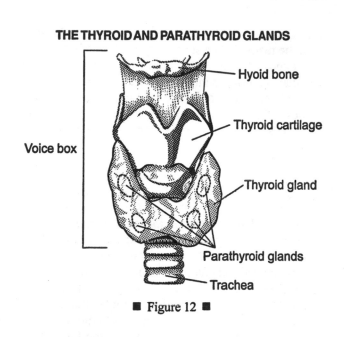

■ Figure 12 ■

The Integumentary System

The **integumentary system,** better known as the **skin,** covers the body, and at first glance would not appear to have a direct relationship with nourishment. However, one of its several functions is to prevent water loss. For example, many times a person survives a fire, with severe burns over more than half of his or her body, only to die a few days later from dehydration because too much skin was lost to contain the body's water.

Water loss from the skin, or **perspiration,** is a way of shedding excess heat. People normally perspire when they are warm, as after exercise or on a hot day. The evaporation of perspiration from the skin cools the body. When it's cold, blood and the heat it carries are diverted away from skin. Perspiration also carries salt (sodium chloride) from the body. Consequently, a person who has perspired freely may have to replace salt as well as water, although most diets normally contain enough salt to replace what is lost.

The skin can be important in the production of **vitamin D.** This nutrient can be made from a sterol, a derivative of cholesterol, when the skin is exposed to sunlight. The sunlight alters the sterol to a compound that is absorbed into the blood and then converted to vitamin D by the liver. Skin exposed to sunlight makes as much vitamin D as the body needs; it never produces an overdose. However, overexposure to the sun has other consequences, such as skin cancer.

The Muscular System

The **muscular system** is perhaps the most massive system in the body, and it may be the greatest single consumer of energy. Muscles consume large amounts of sugar and fat, and they need protein in order to be maintained and produced, although eating massive amounts of protein is not necessary for muscle development. In addition, muscle cells need sodium, potassium, and calcium if they are to function properly. Muscles keep us erect and allow us to move. Consequently, they must do work, and energy nutrients are the fuel for this work. During periods of prolonged starvation, muscle tissue may be cannibalized to provide energy for other organs, such as the brain or the heart. While this condition is not healthy, it can sometimes spell the difference between life and death, provided it does not occur too often or for too long.

The Skeletal System

While the **skeletal system** is generally thought to include only the **bones,** it also includes the **joints,** the connections between the bones, and the tissues involved in those connections. However, the bones are the most critical part of the skeletal system in terms of nutrition because of their need for the mineral **calcium.** Bones need calcium in order to grow and to maintain and repair themselves. Dietary calcium is deposited on the bones by the action of the hormone **calcitonin,** another hormone produced by the thyroid gland. In addition, the bones serve as the body's reservoir of calcium. When the level of calcium in the blood is low, the parathyroid hormone, parathormone, promotes the absorption of calcium from the intestine, but it also promotes the removal of calcium from the bones if necessary.

The Reproductive System

The **reproductive system** is made up of the organs involved with procreation. In the male, they include the **testes,** which produce sperm cells and male hormones; in the female they include the **ovaries,** which produce egg cells and female hormones, and the **uterus,** where the fetus is carried during pregnancy. The relationship between reproduction and nutrition should be obvious. Bodies that are inadequately nourished often do not have the capacity for reproduction; in particular, inadequately nourished female bodies do not have the means of providing for proper prenatal development; that is, pregnancy will be difficult. A pregnant woman who is poorly nourished may experience deterioration of her own tissues in order to provide nutrients for her developing child. In addition, following birth, adequate nourishment is needed for **lactation,** or milk production. Adequate nutrition is extremely important to reproduction, a topic discussed in more detail on page 170.

Carbohydrates are the fundamental energy nutrient from which all of the other energy nutrients are derived. It is currently recommended that 55% to 75% of our daily caloric intake come from carbohydrates. Carbohydrates are produced by plants initially, and plants are the principal providers of carbohydrates to the human diet. Milk is the only animal-derived food that contains a significant amount of carbohydrate. Carbohydrates provide a significant number of calories for most of the animals we eat and a significant amount of our own energy. For some activities, such as strength-requiring work, and some parts of our bodies, such as our nervous systems, carbohydrates are the principal, preferred, and perhaps only source of energy.

Monosaccharides: The Simple Sugars

The basic carbohydrate is the compound **glucose** (Figure 13), the building block from which all other carbohydrates are made. Glucose is arranged with five of its six carbon atoms and one oxygen atom forming a ring. The orientation of the hydrogen atoms and hydroxyl (OH) groups distinguishes glucose from other six-carbon monosaccharides, or **hexoses.**

GLUCOSE ($C_6H_{12}O_6$)

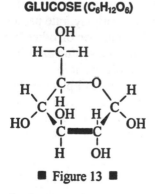

■ Figure 13 ■

Glucose is made in green plants by the process of **photosynthesis,** which works as follows. The green pigment in plants, **chlorophyll,** absorbs sunlight, which it uses to remove hydrogen atoms from six molecules of water. The hydrogen atoms are passed to six molecules of carbon dioxide, and in the rearrangement of hydrogen atoms and carbon dioxide molecules, a molecule of glucose is formed. The oxygen remaining from the water is passed out of the plant. Once the glucose is formed, it can be rearranged to form two additional monosaccharides: **fructose** and **galactose** (Figure 14).

FRUCTOSE AND GALACTOSE

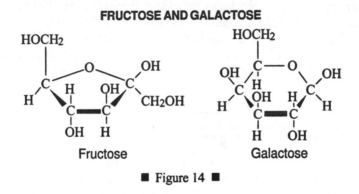

Fructose   Galactose

■ Figure 14 ■

Molecules of both of these sugars contain the same number of carbon, hydrogen, and oxygen atoms as does a molecule of glucose, but the three-dimensional structures of glucose, fructose, and galactose differ. Fructose and galactose are structural **isomers** of glucose. Note that the names of all three carbohydrates mentioned so far end in the letters *-ose.* In fact, carbohydrate names typically end in these three letters. Although a number of other hexose monosaccharides are found in nature or can be synthesized in a laboratory, only glucose, fructose, and galactose are important in human nutrition.

Glucose is typically found in plant materials; corn sweetener is rich in glucose. Fructose tastes sweeter than glucose; it is typically found in fruit and in honey. Galactose is never found alone in nature; rather, it is always linked to a glucose molecule (as described in the discussion of lactose below).

Disaccharides

Sucrose. By definition, a **disaccharide** is made up of two linked monosaccharides. The most common of these is **sucrose,** better known as table sugar or cane sugar. It is composed of a molecule of glucose and a molecule of fructose (Figure 15). Table sugar is typically refined from sugar cane or from sugar beets, but the compound is common in many vegetables and in fruits.

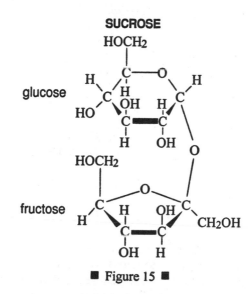

■ Figure 15 ■

Refined sucrose is routinely used in desserts, candy, and other frequently consumed sweets, and it is sometimes added to other foods to enhance flavor. Nutritionally, however, there is a vast difference between eating refined sucrose in desserts and eating natural sucrose in fruits and vegetables. Fruits and vegetables are nutrient dense, providing such nutrients as fiber (discussed later in this chapter), vitamins, and minerals, in addition to sugar. In contrast, foods made with refined sucrose often contain little more than sugar and provide only energy.

Lactose. Lactose is commonly known as **milk sugar** because it is found in milk, the only animal-derived food that contains significant amounts of carbohydrate. A cup of cow's milk typically contains 12 grams; a cup of human milk contains roughly 19 grams. Lactose consists of a molecule of glucose bonded to a molecule of galactose (Figure 16). Milk is a baby's first food and a major part of the diet throughout infancy and early childhood. The lactose in milk provides a child with much of the energy needed for growth and development.

LACTOSE

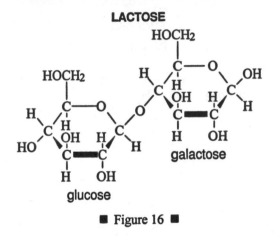

■ Figure 16 ■

Occasionally, one hears of a person who is allergic to milk. Usually, the allergy is not to lactose but to one of the milk proteins. However, sugar in milk gives some people problems. One disorder is **galactosemia,** a hereditary condition in which the enzyme necessary for the metabolism of galactose is lacking. To have this disorder, one must inherit a gene for it from *both* parents. Neither of the parents need have the disorder, but both must carry it, at the very least. Carriers inherit the gene from only one parent, not both. Children with galactosemia must drink a milk substitute with a digestible carbohydrate if they are to develop normally. Another condition, **lactose intolerance,** develops with age. A person with the condition was born able to produce the intestinal enzyme **lactase** (necessary to split lactose into glucose and galactose), but he or she later loses the ability. Sometimes the onset of lactose intolerance occurs in adulthood, sometimes in childhood, but it usually develops when milk is no longer critical for survival.

If a lactose-intolerant individual drinks milk, or perhaps eats a milk product like ice cream, the lactose passes through the small intestine and into the large intestine. There it is attacked by bacteria, which ferment the sugar, giving off gas in the process. The gas can cause discomfort or, worse, severe cramping, along with flatulence and diarrhea. People at risk of lactose intolerance are typically of Asian, African, Native American, or Semitic ancestry. Fortunately for the lactose intolerant, one can now buy the enzyme in pill form and take it whenever dairy products are consumed.

Maltose. Maltose and its isomer **isomaltose** (Figure 17) are nutritionally more important as components of polysaccharides (discussed below) than they are as disaccharides. Both maltose and isomaltose consist of two glucose molecules. They differ, however, in that maltose is formed by a bond between the first carbon of one glucose molecule and the fourth carbon of the second, while isomaltose is formed by a bond between the first carbon of one molecule and the sixth carbon of the other.

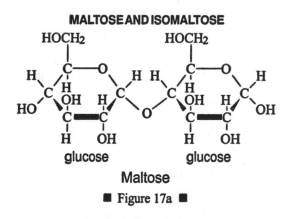

MALTOSE AND ISOMALTOSE

Maltose

■ Figure 17a ■

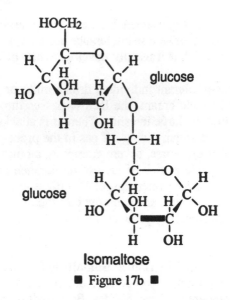

Isomaltose

■ Figure 17b ■

Another isomer of maltose is the disaccharide **cellobiose** (Figure 18). It differs from maltose in the bonding angle between the two glucose molecules. Cellobiose also is more important as a component of polysaccharides than it is as a disaccharide. It cannot be digested by humans.

CELLOBIOSE

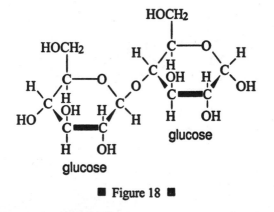

■ Figure 18 ■

Polysaccharides

Sometimes referred to as **complex carbohydrates,** the **polysaccharides** are derived from disaccharides. They are composed of many glucose units linked in long chains, sometimes branched, sometimes not. Two types of polysaccharides are important in human nutrition: starches and plant fibers. A third important polysaccharide, one that is produced by the body, not eaten, is the compound glycogen, which is the storage form of glucose in human tissue.

Glycogen. Only a small amount of carbohydrate is stored in human tissue, mostly in the liver and muscles. All dietary carbohydrate is eventually converted or reduced to glucose, and that which is not used immediately is stored as **glycogen,** highly branched chains of glucose molecules. Liver glycogen is slowly broken down to maintain blood glucose at a nearly constant level. In muscles, glycogen is used to provide the glucose needed for exercise.

Starch. Like glycogen, **starch** is initially derived from maltose and isomaltose, and it consists of many linked glucose molecules. Starch chains are less highly branched than are glycogen chains, and some types are not branched at all. Plants typically store energy as starch. Annual plants, like corn, have starchy seeds to provide an energy source for young plants. Starch is stored in structures such as bulbs or tubers (for example, potatoes) that provide energy to perennial, soft-stemmed plants when they sprout in the spring.

Grains, such as wheat, corn, and rice, are the principal dietary source of starch in much of the world and the single greatest source of calories in human nutrition. For many years, people incorrectly believed that calories from starchy foods were more likely to cause obesity than were calories from other foods. Currently, however, it is believed that Americans should increase the amount of starch they eat. U.S. government guidelines now suggest eating 6 to 11 servings of grains each day.

Fiber. Fiber, derived from cellobiose, makes up most of the structural parts of plants. It is composed principally of the polysaccharide **cellulose,** but it also includes other polysaccharides such as **pectin** and **hemicellulose.** Plants make fiber by first making cellobiose, not maltose as they do in starch production. Fiber is indigestible. The bonding angle between glucose molecules in cellobiose, and therefore in fiber, does not allow fiber to fit into human digestive enzymes. Perhaps the most familiar source of fiber is **bran,** the covering of the seed within the inedible husk. However, most plant materials that are eaten, unless they are severely refined, contain fiber, and people who lack fiber in their diets are simply eating too few fruits, vegetables, and whole grains.

Fiber may be classified as soluble or insoluble. Most plant foods contain mixtures of the two, but some, like wheat bran or brown rice, tend to be rich in insoluble fiber, while others, like oat bran and rye, tend to be rich in soluble fiber.

The consumption of **insoluble fiber** has been linked with the health of the large intestine. In particular, it maintains the function of the large intestine by absorbing water and providing a bulky mass for the large intestine to push on, which prevents its cramping and exercises its muscles, promoting the health of the organ. Furthermore, insoluble fiber helps in preventing constipation, hemorrhoids, and diverticulitis and may help to protect against colon cancer as well. Insoluble fiber regulates bowel movements and softens stools, making them easier to eliminate. In addition, the fiber may bind potentially carcinogenic (cancer causing) chemicals and speed their removal from the body, in this way possibly preventing other cancers.

Soluble fiber slows the movement of food through the stomach and upper digestive tract, which promotes a feeling of fullness and staves off hunger. It also slows the absorption of glucose, which keeps blood sugar levels higher for longer periods and further staves off hunger. This blood sugar regulation is especially important to diabetics (see below). Furthermore, soluble fiber is thought to help reduce the risk of heart disease by lowering blood cholesterol levels. Bile from the liver contains cholesterol which is normally reabsorbed and recycled into the blood. Soluble fiber binds bile and prevents its recycling. Furthermore, it may also bind dietary fat, which is converted to blood cholesterol by the liver.

One way in which both types of fiber can reduce the risk of heart disease and possibly contribute to weight reduction (or at least prevent weight gain) is by displacing high-fat and calorie-dense foods from the diet. However, a high-fiber diet has some drawbacks. Since fiber absorbs water and carries it out of the body, it can lead to dehydration if sufficient water is not consumed. In addition, if adequate water is not present, some fibers can harden the stool and cause intestinal blockage. While fiber may bind possible carcinogens, it also can bind certain minerals, such as iron, calcium, and zinc, and carry them out of the body, possibly leading to deficiencies. Some fibers are also capable of being fermented by intestinal bacteria, thus causing flatulence.

Digestion and Regulation of Carbohydrates

The body's principal use of carbohydrates is for energy, particularly short-term energy. In order to use carbohydrates, the body must first reduce them to monosaccharides, a process accomplished by the digestive system.

The first action on carbohydrates is by the enzyme **salivary amylase,** which is secreted by the salivary glands and begins digesting starch in the mouth. (Partial breakdown of some starches, such as that in vegetables, is accomplished by cooking.) No action on carbohydrates occurs in the stomach, but in the small intestine, enzymes complete the breakdown of disaccharides to monosaccharides, which are then absorbed into the blood. All hexose isomers are converted to glucose in the liver.

Blood from the intestines is carried to the liver. There, glucose is absorbed and converted to glycogen under the influence of the pancreatic hormone **insulin.** Insulin promotes the uptake of glucose and its conversion to glycogen in the muscles as well, and it may promote the conversion of excess glucose to fat. This regulation keeps the blood glucose level from getting too high. As the various tissues remove glucose from the blood to satisfy their energy needs, blood glucose level drops. In response, the pancreas secretes a second hormone, **glucagon,** which promotes the breakdown of glycogen in the liver to glucose and its subsequent release into the blood. This regulation keeps the blood glucose level from getting too low, thus protecting body proteins from being cannibalized for energy (see the chapter beginning on page 87). Because there is only a finite amount of glycogen in the liver, however, blood sugar eventually falls below the critical level, a condition recognized as hunger.

Getting Energy from Sugar

The energy in sugar is stored within the chemical bonds of the molecule, and it can be released only by breaking those bonds, a process accomplished inside cells through the action of a number of enzymes. The energy in sugar is used to produce a cellular compound called **adenosine triphosphate (ATP)** from two normal cell constituents, **adenosine diphosphate (ADP)** and **phosphoric acid.** Some of the energy required to combine ADP and phosphoric acid is held by the ATP molecule in a **high-energy bond;** when that bond is broken, energy is released for cell functions, such as muscle contraction. The removal of energy from glucose occurs in three stages: glycolysis, the Krebs cycle, and electron transport.

Glycolysis. The first stage of glucose breakdown, **glycolysis,** occurs in the cytoplasm of the cell. Here, the six-carbon molecule goes through a series of steps to become two three-carbon molecules called **pyruvic acid.** Because glucose is a stable compound, some energy must be added to it to start the breakdown process, analogous perhaps to the energy required in striking a match to make it light. Two molecules of ATP are sacrificed to provide this energy, but replacements for those two plus two more are generated in the breakdown of glucose to pyruvic acid.

The Krebs cycle. Once pyruvic acid has formed, it is carried into a mitochondrion where it reacts with a carrier molecule called **coenzyme A.** The reaction releases a molecule of carbon dioxide from the pyruvic acid. It diffuses from the cell and is carried by the blood to the lungs, where it is exhaled. The remaining two-carbon fragment goes through another series of reactions in which the remaining carbons are lost as carbon dioxide and the hydrogen atoms, which carry the bulk of the molecule's energy, are passed to hydrogen acceptors. (Some hydrogen atoms are released during glycolysis too, and these are also passed to hydrogen acceptors, which carry them into the mitochondrion.) A single molecule of ATP is generated by the passage of each pyruvic acid molecule through the **Krebs cycle;** however, a number of hydrogen atoms remain to be dealt with, which occurs in the next stage.

Electron transport. The hydrogen atoms, still inside the mitochondrion, are passed through a series of acceptors. In this series, the lion's share of ATP molecules are produced, but at the end, the hydrogen atoms must be removed because too much hydrogen in a cell alters the chemical environment and can interfere with many cellular processes. Oxygen that was inhaled into the lungs and transported by the blood to the tissues reacts with the hydrogen atoms to produce water. The hydrogen is safely eliminated as water in the urinary system.

Problems with Sugar

Diabetes. The regulation of blood sugar level is an important function in the use of carbohydrates. It is accomplished by the hormones insulin and glucagon, both of which are produced by structures in the pancreas called the **islets of Langerhans** or **pancreatic islets.** In some people, however, the production or effectiveness of insulin is compromised, resulting in the condition known as **diabetes mellitus.** The two types of this disease are insulin dependent diabetes (IDDM) and noninsulin dependent diabetes (NIDDM) (or Type I and Type II, respectively).

Insulin dependent (Type I) diabetes is the less common of the two, affecting from 10% to 20% of all diabetics. No one is certain of the cause of this disease, but some researchers now think that it has a hereditary root and is initiated by an environmental trigger, perhaps a virus. Type I diabetes appears to be an **autoimmune disorder** in which the body attacks the pancreatic islets as if they were invading organisms and destroys their insulin-producing capability. To replace pancreatic insulin, insulin dependent diabetics must take insulin injections every day so that the glucose from the carbohydrate they consume can be converted to glycogen. (Insulin is a protein; if it were taken orally, it would be digested.)

Without insulin, glucose accumulates in the blood, and the body's only way to return the blood sugar level to normal is through removal of glucose by the kidneys. But in this removal process, the glucose carries water with it, The elimination of glucose in this way can lead to dehydration and one of the symptoms of diabetes, excessive thirst. Furthermore, because no glucose has been stored, when normal demands remove glucose from the blood and drop the level below its critical minimum, there is no glycogen to tap to replace it. To meet energy needs, the body taps fat reserves, but without glucose present, the fat cannot be used properly. Instead it forms **ketone bodies** (Figure 19), fragments of fat that are rich in energy but potentially toxic. (The compound that gives airplane glue its characteristic odor is a ketone body, and a diabetic may have breath that has a similar smell.) The combination of dehydration and **ketosis** can upset diabetics' internal chemistry so much that it can cause passing out. Some diabetics do not find out about their condition until they've been taken unconscious to a hospital. If diabetes is not treated, coma and death are possible.

A KETONE (ACETONE)

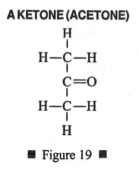

■ Figure 19 ■

Noninsulin dependent (Type II) diabetes is more clearly hereditary than is insulin dependent diabetes, and it usually begins after the age of forty. In this type of diabetes, insulin is produced, but it is ineffective because body cells resist its action. The Type II diabetic has problems similar to those of the Type I diabetic (including the possibility of coma), except ketosis, but cannot control them with insulin injections. Type II diabetes is treated primarily through diet and weight control. By avoiding simple sugars, Type II diabetics can prevent blood sugar surges, and by controlling their weight, they are able to keep their insulin more effective. When these measures do not control the problem, oral drugs that increase the effectiveness of insulin can be used.

A third, uncommon type of diabetes is **gestational diabetes.** As the name suggests, it affects pregnant women. Overweight women and those with a family history of diabetes are most at risk. Usually, the condition is temporary and glucose regulation returns to normal following delivery.

Hypoglycemia. Hypoglycemia is a condition in which the blood glucose level is low (*hypo* means *under*), below the critical level. The condition occurs in diabetics who have taken too much insulin. In nondiabetics, a form of the condition called **reactive hypoglycemia** can occur a few hours after eating a meal that is high in simple sugars. Another form of hypoglycemia, sometimes called **fasting hypoglycemia,** may occur when an individual goes without eating for an extended period. Hypoglycemia also can be triggered by pancreatic damage such as a tumor or cancer or by liver disease, but in general, hypoglycemia is rare.

Tooth decay. Described in an earlier chapter, **tooth decay,** or **dental caries,** can result from the accumulation of carbohydrates on the teeth and the resulting breakdown of those carbohydrates by oral bacteria. The acid waste products of the bacteria erode the tooth enamel and allow bacteria to infect the softer dentin beneath. Simple sugars may not be the biggest villains in this problem, however, because they are highly soluble and easily washed off the teeth with water or even saliva. Glucose and fructose are less cariogenic than sucrose. Complex carbohydrates, like starch, may be the greater problem because they tend to stick to the teeth more than the simple sugars. Other factors come into play, however, including the hardness of the teeth, the nature of the bacteria (some people have more cariogenic bacteria in their mouths than others), the quality of tooth care, and factors in the diet (foods like cheese, peanuts, and apples appear to prevent tooth decay, as does fluoride in drinking water).

Obesity. In theory, **obesity** results from consuming more calories than are used. The excess food is converted to fat and stored. For many years, carbohydrates were thought to be the principal contributors to obesity, and dieters were told to avoid starchy foods like bread and potatoes. More recently, evidence has suggested that it is dietary fat, not carbohydrates, that contributes to obesity and that diets high in carbohydrates, particularly complex carbohydrates, but low in fat do not promote obesity, especially if the carbohydrates come from fruits and vegetables.

Behavior. For years, sugar was thought to be a cause of **hyperactivity** in children. However, recent research has shown that this is not the case. In fact, sugar may even have a calming effect because it promotes the production of **serotonin,** a brain chemical that promotes sleep.

Sugar Substitutes

Because of misconceptions about the role of carbohydrates, including sugar, in obesity and behavior, because consumers wish to reduce their overall calorie intake, and because they can be of benefit to diabetics, **sugar substitutes** have had a ready market. Those that provide sweetness without providing calories are known as **nonnutritive sweeteners.**

Polyols (sugar alcohols). Three common polyols are **mannitol, sorbitol,** and **xylitol.** They contain roughly half as many calories as sucrose, so they cannot be considered nonnutritive sweeteners. However, they may not be as readily absorbed as glucose and fructose; consequently, their sweetness can be enjoyed without great concern about calories. Oral bacteria do not metabolize some of the polyols, making them safe additives for sugarless gums. However, some intestinal bacteria can ferment polyols, and if one consumes too much, intestinal distress can follow.

Aspartame. Better known by its commercial names **NutraSweet** and **Equal, aspartame** is roughly as caloric as sugar but two hundred times sweeter. Therefore, only minute amounts are required to provide a lot of sweetening. NutraSweet contains the amino acids **aspartic acid** and **phenylalanine.** This sweetener has been researched extensively and found safe for consumption by both children and adults. The phenylalanine does pose a risk for people with the hereditary condition **phenylketonuria (PKU),** described on page 102, but phenylalanine is found in virtually all foods. For example, a glass of milk has six times as much phenylalanine as a glass of diet soda sweetened with aspartame. Another suggested drawback of aspartame is that when it's digested in the intestine, it yields methyl alcohol. Again, however, many other foods, like tomato juice, contain it. In general, research suggests that aspartame is perfectly safe to use.

Saccharin. Saccharin is the oldest of the sugar substitutes and is entirely nonnutritive. It is not broken down in the digestive system, it does not promote tooth decay, and it is readily eliminated from the body. Saccharin is 50% sweeter than an equal amount of sugar but has a somewhat bitter aftertaste. It was found to be weakly carcinogenic in rats, and the Food and Drug Administration proposed banning it in 1977. Usually, any food that has been found to cause cancer in laboratory animals cannot be sold in the United States for human consumption. However, because no cases of human cancer have been related to saccharin and because it has been important to people on sugar-restricted diets, such as diabetics, especially before the appearance of the other sugar substitutes, continued use of the product was allowed but with a warning on labels of saccharin-containing products. In general, it seems that people do not consume saccharin in dangerous quantities.

Lipids are a collection of organic (carbon- and hydrogen-containing) compounds that are soluble in organic solvents, such as alcohol or chloroform, but have limited soulubility in water. Characteristically, the ratio of carbon to hydrogen in lipids is roughly one to two. They also contain oxygen, but much less abundantly. It is convenient to divide the lipids into two subcategories: fats and sterols.

Fats

Fats are energy nutrients; in fact, they are the most concentrated form of energy available in the diet. Each gram of fat contains about nine calories, more than twice the number in an equal amount of carbohydrate or protein. Fats not only provide calories for immediate use but also are the form in which excess calories provided by fats and other nutrients are stored in the body. It is convenient to subdivide the fats into two groups: glycerides and phospholipids. **Glycerides** and **phospholipids** have different biological functions, and some nutrition scientists suggest that glycerides, sterols, and phospholipids are all equal-level subcategories of lipids. However, chemically, glycerides and phospholipids are quite similar, as discussed below. Informally, you may hear the term *fat* used to describe those glycerides that are solid at room temperature and the term *oils* used to describe those that are liquid at room temperature. However, both are correctly described by the broad, more technical term fat.

Glycerides. All **glycerides** are combinations of a three-carbon carbohydrate, **glycerol** (Figure 20a) and from one to three **fatty acids.** Glycerides that contain a single fatty acid are **monoglycerides;** those with two fatty acids are **diglycerides** (Figure 20b); and those with three fatty acids are **triglycerides** (Figure 20c). Virtually all fats in the diet are triglycerides, as are the fats that are stored in the body.

GLYCEROL AND GLYCERIDES

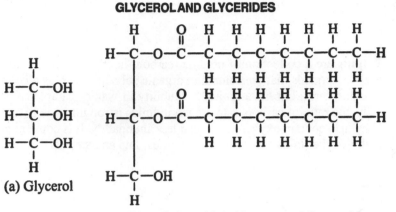

(a) Glycerol

(b) A diglyceride with saturated fatty acids

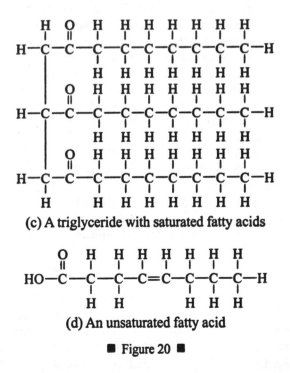

(c) A triglyceride with saturated fatty acids

(d) An unsaturated fatty acid

■ Figure 20 ■

Fatty acids are constructed from hydrocarbons, but they have a **carboxyl group** at one end of the molecule. The carbon atom that is closest to the carboxyl group is called the **alpha carbon;** the one farthest away—that is, at the other end of the hydrocarbon chain—is the **omega carbon** (see Figure 22, p.76). Fatty acids vary in the number of carbons in the chain, but the number is always even.

If the interior carbon atoms in the fatty acid chain are each linked to two hydrogen atoms and the omega carbon is linked to three hydrogen atoms, the fatty acid is said to be a **saturated fatty acid** (Figure 20b and 20c). In a saturated fatty acid, every site on a carbon atom that can be occupied by a hydrogen atom is so occupied (the carbon atom is "saturated" with hydrogen atoms), and adjacent carbons share only a single pair of electrons (single bond), with each of the other pair being shared with a hydrogen atom.

In contrast, in an **unsaturated fatty acid** (Figure 20d), at least two adjacent carbon atoms form a **double bond** (p. 17); that is, they share two pairs of electrons. An unsaturated fatty acid that contains only one point of unsaturation (double bond between adjacent carbon atoms) is described as a **monounsaturated fatty acid,** sometimes referred to as a *mufa* fatty acid. A fatty acid that contains two or more points of unsaturation is called a **polyunsaturated fatty acid** (*pufa* fatty acid).

Saturated fats typically contain only saturated fatty acids, are solid at room temperature, and come from foods of animal origin. **Unsaturated fats** contain at least one unsaturated fatty acid. **Polyunsaturated fats** contain at least one polyunsaturated fatty acid or there are several points of unsaturation among the three fatty acids they contain. Polyunsaturated fats are typically liquid at room temperature and are from foods of plant origin.

Phospholipids. Phospholipids (Figure 21) are similar in structure to triglycerides, but rather than having three fatty acids bonded to glycerol, they have only two plus a molecule of a compound containing a phosphate group ($H_2PO_4^+$). Phospholipids are structural molecules, components of cell membranes.

LECITHIN, A PHOSPHOLIPID

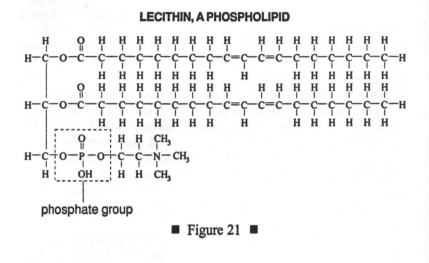

phosphate group

■ Figure 21 ■

Functions of Fat

Fat is efficient in **energy storage.** In earlier times, the ability to store fat on their bodies may have allowed our ancestors to survive periods when little food was available. Because fats are more energy dense than are carbohydrates, the volume of stored fat is much smaller than the volume of carbohydrate containing an equal number of calories. In addition to storing energy, fat is also an **immediate source of energy** for some parts of the body, particularly the muscular system. There are two types of voluntary muscles: red and white, which weight lifters refer to as slow-twitch and quick-twitch muscles, respectively. Red muscle, which is used for endurance activities, such as long-distance running, burns fat, as does the heart, which is made of muscle similar to red muscle.

Fat also provides **protection** for some of the body's organs. The kidneys, in particular, are protected by a padding of fat that helps to hold them in place and cushion impacts that could otherwise injure them. In addition, people, especially women, carry a layer of fat under the skin, which helps to **insulate** the body against cold temperatures.

Finally, fat in food serves a number of dietary functions. Fat in the stomach slows down its emptying and provides a feeling of fullness, of **satiety.** (Traditional Chinese cooking—not necessarily the food served in American "Chinese" restaurants—is low in fat, which may account for its reputation of leaving one hungry an hour after eating.) Fat in food also provides **flavor.** A plain baked potato, which many people find bland, contains virtually no fat. However, even a small amount of fat in the form of butter or sour cream enhances the taste of the potato considerably. In addition, fat aids in the **absorption of fat-soluble vitamins** and some **minerals** in the small intestine.

Dietary Sources of Fat

Because of the linkage of fat intake (particularly the intake of saturated fat) and health problems in recent years (discussed below, pp. 81–85), it is important to distinguish the types of fats in the diet in order to plan to reduce the consumption of those that are less desirable.

The principal natural sources of saturated fat in the diet are animal foods: **meats** and **dairy products.** In many dairy products, such as homogenized milk and most cheeses, fat is blended with, and difficult to separate from, the product. Other dairy products, such as butter and sour cream, are essentially pure fat. In choice cuts of red meat, fat is marbled through the meat and cannot be efficiently removed, while in cheaper cuts, it's often concentrated along the side and is more easily trimmed away.

Poultry and **fish fats,** especially fish fat, are typically less saturated, less integrated into the meat, and more easily removed than those of red meat. The diets of North Americans, however, include a great deal of red meat.

In general, **plants** are far less rich in fats than are animals. In addition, plant fats are typically **unsaturated fats,** are liquid at room temperature (oils), and are usually extracted from seeds. Three plant fats are notable exceptions to the generality that plant fats are unsat-

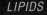

urated. **Palm oil, palm kernel oil,** and **coconut oil** are among the most highly saturated fats in nature.

In North America, a large quantity of fat is added to food during processing and preparation. For example, butter or lard is typically used for frying, and beef fat (saturated fat technically known as tallow) has been used historically for deep-frying (immersing foods into boiling fat). Much restaurant food, especially the fast-food fare so popular with North Americans, such as French fries, is prepared in this way. Fortunately, many restaurants have recently switched to less saturated fats in their food preparation.

North Americans are also fond of sweet snacks and desserts. Cookies and cakes are very rich in fat, which is added to enhance their flavor. Food flavorings and condiments, such as butter, sour cream, and mayonnaise, add much fat to the diet, and certain popular foods that essentially masquerade as meat, such as hotdogs and bacon, are actually little more than fat.

The Body's Handling of Fat

The digestion and absorption of fat. Dietary fat is little affected by chemical digestion in the mouth or stomach. However, the arrival of partly digested material from the stomach into the small intestine triggers the contraction of the gallbladder, which discharges **liver bile** into the small intestine where it emulsifies fats to aid in their digestion. In the small intestine, the pancreatic enzyme **lipase** breaks down triglycerides to monoglycerides and fatty acids.

The products of fat digestion are absorbed through the intestinal wall, but only the smallest fatty acids are absorbed directly into the blood. The remaining products of fat digestion are combined with protein and cholesterol for transport through the lymphatic system, from which they eventually enter the blood by way of the large thoracic duct, which empties into the subclavian vein that drains the arm.

The body's use of fat. Some fat is used immediately, as is carbohydrate, to fuel the heart and the red voluntary muscles. The products of the digested fat react with oxygen, liberating energy, in the mitochondria (as described on p. 25). Fat that is not used immediately is stored. In men, storage is typically in the chest and midsection, around the intestines, and even around the heart. In women, fat is more typically stored in the breasts and on the hips, buttocks, and thighs. In terms of health, the female pattern of fat deposition is much preferable to that of the male.

When calorie intake is less than calories used, the body turns to its fat deposits to make up the difference. In theory, when too few calories are eaten, the body should burn fat and lose weight. However, as is discussed in the chapter on weight control (p. 135), it is not quite that simple. The central nervous system can burn only carbohydrate, not fat, and fat cannot be converted to carbohydrate. Consequently, if too little carbohydrate is eaten, the body turns to protein—muscles and organs—rather than fat to make up the difference for this system. When it does, the rate of metabolism, that is, the rate at which the body burns calories, slows down. To a dieter who has cut down drastically on his or her calorie intake to lose weight, this situation is counterproductive and frustrating.

Essential fatty acids. The body can synthesize fat from excess protein or carbohydrate, manufacturing both the glycerol and the fatty acids. In fact, the body can produce virtually all of the fat it needs. However, the body produces only saturated fatty acids but requires two unsaturated fatty acids, linolenic acid and linoleic acid (Figure 22), for synthesis of a number of regulatory compounds. These fatty acids function with lecithin (a phospholipid) in cell membranes. Since they cannot be synthesized, they must be consumed and consequently are described as **essential fatty acids.** A diet inadequate in these compounds will eventually lead to deficiencies. Evidence of deficiencies includes liver and kidney disorders and skin problems. Long-term deficiencies can cause reproductive failures, and deficiencies in childhood can cause growth retardation.

Linolenic acid is known as an **omega-3 unsaturated fatty acid,** that is, one in which the first point of unsaturation is found between the third and fourth carbons from the omega carbon, counting the omega (terminal) carbon as the first one (Figure 22a). Linolenic acid is found in seafood, particularly in the oils of cold-water marine fishes, like salmon. Greenland and Alaskan Inuit, who eat such fish abundantly, have very low rates of heart disease, in spite of the large amounts of saturated fat that they consume. (The role of saturated fat in heart disease is discussed beginning on p. 83.) Research has indicated that omega-3 unsaturated fatty acids play a role in avoiding heart disease, but supplements of these fatty acids have not proved to offer the protection that eating oily fish does. Linolenic acid can also be found in vegetable oils and some leafy green vegetables, although in lesser amounts.

Linoleic acid is an **omega-6 unsaturated fatty acid,** one in which the first point of unsaturation occurs between the sixth and seventh carbons from the omega carbon (Figure 22b). Linoleic acid is found in poultry, eggs, leafy vegetables, and seeds, oils, nuts, and grains.

LINOLENIC AND LINOLEIC ACID

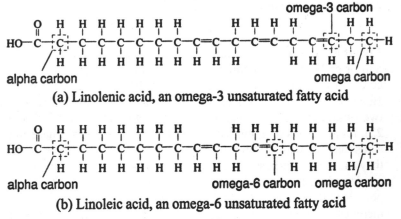

(a) Linolenic acid, an omega-3 unsaturated fatty acid

(b) Linoleic acid, an omega-6 unsaturated fatty acid

■ Figure 22 ■

Preservation of Fats

Saturated fats and fatty acids are stable compounds, but the points of unsaturation in unsaturated fats are vulnerable to reaction with oxygen and reactive chemicals called **free radicals**. Such reactions are usually referred to as **oxidations**. Oxidative damage can occur to fats in cell membranes and can possibly lead to cancer or heart disease. Oxidation can also occur in unsaturated fats in foods or in cooking oil, spoiling them, or making them rancid.

Sealing and refrigeration. One method of preventing oxidation is keeping the oil **isolated** from oxygen, which can be as easy as keeping the oil in a tightly sealed container. Another means of prevention is keeping the oil **refrigerated** because chemical reactions are retarded at lower temperatures. More sophisticated methods include the use of preservatives and hydrogenation.

Preservatives. **Preservatives** are chemical compounds that are so named because they are added to food to preserve freshness. The preservatives used with unsaturated fats are known as **antioxidants.** They essentially compete with unsaturated fats for the oxygen and free radicals that could break the points of unsaturation. By becoming oxidized themselves, the antioxidants prevent the unsaturated fat from becoming oxidized.

The two most frequently used preservatives are known by their three-letter abbreviations: **BHT** (butylated hydroxytoluene) and **BHA** (butylated hydroxyanisole). These compounds have been falsely maligned as carcinogens. There is no evidence to indicate that they are in any way harmful in the concentrations used in foods. Natural antioxidants also exist and include vitamins A, C, and E.

Hydrogenation. Hydrogenation is accomplished by adding **hydrogen.** When an unsaturated fat or fatty acid is hydrogenated, the compound becomes saturated and solidified. Certain vegetable shortenings are essentially hydrogenated oils. Unsaturated peanut oil is routinely hydrogenated in the manufacture of peanut butter, which not only preserves the peanut oil, but also keeps the peanut butter homogenized. In so-called natural peanut butter, in which the oil is not hydrogenated, the oil and peanuts separate from one another and must be blended before the peanut butter can be used.

Sometimes, oils are **partially hydrogenated,** which means that they are treated with enough hydrogen to break some of the points of unsaturation, but not all. Partial hydrogenation is also a preservation technique. It is used in foods such as stuffing mixes and snack crackers. This practice can possibly lead to problems because of changes it can make in the shape of the fatty acid molecule. Fatty acids are normally helically coiled (spiral) molecules. They straighten out at points of unsaturation, but the rest of the molecule remains coiled. If the plane (in the mathematical sense) of the point of unsaturation is thought of as a dividing line between two hemispheres, in naturally occurring unsaturated fatty acids, the coiled fragments of the molecule on either side of the point of unsaturation are always in the same hemisphere, either above or below the plane of the point of unsaturation. This is called the **cis** configuration, and naturally occurring unsaturated fatty acids are **cis-fatty acids** (Figure 23a). However, if two points of unsaturation exist in a single fatty acid molecule and only one of them is broken by partial hydrogenation, the resulting, still unsaturated, molecule may end up with the coiled fragments on either side of the point of saturation in opposite hemispheres. This is called a **trans** configuration, and the fatty acid that results is referred to as a **trans-fatty acid** (Figure 23b). If **trans-fatty acids** are eaten, they can be incorporated into cell membranes and affect their functioning. It has been suggested that trans-fatty acids are involved in cancer and heart disease, although exactly how they are involved is not known.

A CIS-FATTY ACID AND A TRANS-FATTY ACID

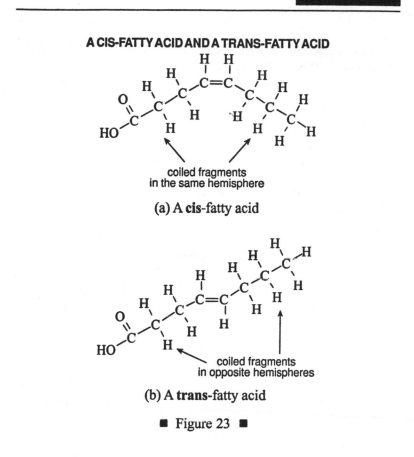

(a) A **cis**-fatty acid

(b) A **trans**-fatty acid

■ Figure 23 ■

Emulsification

A number of foods, such as salad dressings, are made with oil that could separate from the other, water-based, components of the product. Solving the problem with hydrogenation, as is used with peanut butter, is not an option with these foods if they must remain liquid. Manufacturers solve this problem by using **emulsifiers,** compounds that are soluble in both oil and watter and consequently allow the two to mix. Emulsifiers work essentially the same way that bile does on fats that have been eaten; they break the fat into small globules that can be dispersed in the water-based compounds. A common emulsifier is the phospholipid **lecithin** (Figure 21).

Sterols

Sterols, sometimes called **steroids,** are large, complex molecules that contain a skeleton of four hydrocarbon rings. The best-known sterol is **cholesterol** (Figure 24), probably because of its role in heart disease (discussed beginning on p. 83). Cholesterol is, however, important in many body functions.

CHOLESTEROL

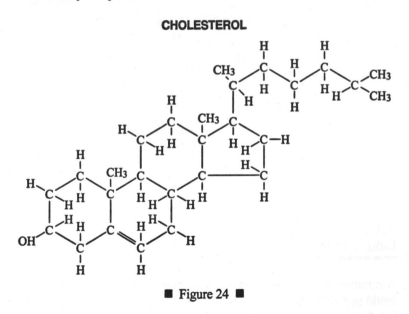

■ Figure 24 ■

Compounds such as vitamin D in the skin, the steroid hormones in the adrenal glands, and the reproductive hormones in the gonads are made from cholesterol. Because it is simultaneously soluble in water and in organic solvents, it can transport fat throughout the blood. The cholesterol associated with this transport is actually a combination of cholesterol, fat, and protein and is referred to as **lipoprotein.** The three cholesterol-containing lipoproteins are **low density lipoprotein (LDL cholesterol), very low density lipoprotein (VLDL cholesterol),** and **high density lipoprotein (HDL cholesterol).**

In addition to transporting fats in the blood, cholesterol is important in their digestion. Cholesterol is a principal component of **liver bile,** generally referred to simply as **bile.** When the bile is released into the duodenum and mixes with partially digested food released from the stomach, it emulsifies the fat, that is, breaks it into tiny globules that can be suspended in water and attacked by fat-digesting enzymes.

There is a fourth category of lipoprotein, the **chylomicrons,** which do not contain cholesterol. Chylomicrons are clusters of protein and products of lipid digestion. They help in the transport of fat in the blood.

Problems with Fats and Cholesterol

Obesity. Virtually everybody is aware that, in most people, excessive body fat is a result of chronic overeating, that is, the consumption of more calories than are used. But other factors can contribute to the production of body fat, including hereditary tendency.

For much of human history, the ability to produce body fat has been critical to survival. Our ancestors often had to face seasonal periods of low food availability, for example, during a long, cold winter or a prolonged dry season. Gaining weight during the summer or rainy season, when food was abundant, was critical to surviving the lean period. Our bodies retain the ability to store energy in this way, even though in modern society such storage is often less critical than it has been in the past, and if the stored energy is not used, it accumulates on the body. Even so, fat stores are important, for example to a person who is ill and cannot eat and must rely on them until normal eating patterns resume.

A person whose weight is 10% to 20% greater than his or her ideal body weight is said to be overweight. One who exceeds the ideal weight by more than that is said to be **obese.** Obesity implies that the excess weight a person is carrying is all fat, and it can have a major impact on health. Obesity has been linked with heart disease, diabetes, gallbladder disease, and possibly cancer. In addition, obesity aggravates already existing joint problems like arthritis.

Obesity is also a source of social problems. Obese people often have to pay higher life insurance premiums, if they are able to get life insurance at all. Obese people may be social outcasts, and they may be ridiculed, especially if they are children. While it is generally believed that all one has to do to lose weight is to eat less, unfortunately, it's not quite that easy. Ninety-five percent of all dieters gain back the weight they've lost within five years.

Recent studies have shown that weight control is at least partly genetic. Some people have very fine-tuned appetite control; they are able to balance their caloric intake with their caloric expenditure by the efficient regulation of the hypothalamus. Others do not balance their eating and activity quite as precisely; they start to gain weight as their metabolism and activity wane with age. Still others are vulnerable both to how much and to what they eat and can gain weight both by eating too much in general or by eating too much fat in particular. These last two are perhaps the most common scenarios.

Exceptional individuals exist who are able to eat as much as they like without gaining a pound. Their intestines apparently selectively absorb only what they need and disregard the rest. Unfortunately, individuals also exist who seem to gain weight regardless of how careful they are about their eating. Their plight and others are discussed more fully in the chapter beginning on page 135.

Gallbladder disease. The gallbladder, which stores bile as it is produced by the liver, contracts in response to partially digested food in the small intestine and sends the bile into the duodenum to help in the digestion of the fat. Under some conditions, however, chemical reactions can occur within the bile in the gallbladder, forming hard crystals, or **gallstones.** Gallstones can be excruciatingly painful, particularly if the person suffering with them eats something fatty. It is not known what causes gallbladder disease, but it is known that people at greatest risk are typically female, overweight, and over forty.

There are several treatments for gallbladder disease. Careful diet and weight loss are the simplest treatments, but as discussed, losing weight can be difficult, and sticking to a bland diet can be very trying. Medication to dissolve gallstones is available, but once that treatment is begun, a person must continue to take the medication for the rest of his or her life. In many cases, the treatment of choice, and perhaps of last resort, is the surgical removal of the gallbladder, or **cholecystectomy**. Once the gallbladder has been removed, a patient theoretically should follow a low-fat diet. But many physicians advise their patients who have undergone the operation to eat normally.

Heart disease and cholesterol. While cholesterol is an important compound in the body, too much of it has been linked to heart disease and atherosclerosis. For that reason, people with high cholesterol have been advised to limit or avoid it in their diets. But since the body manufactures cholesterol from saturated fat, simply avoiding ingesting cholesterol is not the answer. Saturated fats must be avoided also. Products advertised as being free of cholesterol are often not free of saturated fat. For example, some cookies touted as being cholesterol free have been made with a highly saturated, tropical oil such as palm kernel oil.

LDL cholesterol is generally thought of as the **"bad" cholesterol.** It is generally high in fat, and if its level in the blood gets too high, it can be deposited on artery walls, hardening and narrowing them. This condition is associated with the disease **atherosclerosis,** or hardening of the arteries, and with a number of health risks, particularly heart disease and stroke, as discussed below. VLDL cholesterol contains even more fat than does LDL cholesterol, but it is usually much less abundant in the blood, and it loses triglycerides, perhaps to the body's fat deposits, to become LDL cholesterol. **HDL cholesterol** is often referred to as **"good" cholesterol.** It is low in fat; in fact, it is generated by activities, such as aerobic exercise, that are protective against heart disease.

Cholesterol is measured in milligrams (mg) per deciliter (dl) of blood. (A deciliter is equal to 100 ml or 0.1 L.) In general, total cholesterol levels of 200 mg/dl or less are considered normal. Anything above that level indicates a risk of heart disease. The higher the number, the greater the risk. In addition, ratios of LDL cholesterol to HDL cholesterol of four to one or less are, likewise, considered normal. Ratios greater than this indicate risk.

The processing of cholesterol, like obesity, can be genetically determined. Problems with high cholesterol levels seem to run in certain families. Even with cholesterol-reducing medications, people who have inherited such a tendency may be able to do little or nothing about it. On the other hand, some people have inherited an enviable tendency to maintain a low cholesterol level, regardless of their diets.

A small population in northern Italy has inherited, from an ancestor in whom the gene mutation for the trait occurred, the ability to be unaffected by high blood cholesterol. Research has shown that the French have much less trouble with cholesterol than do Americans, in spite of their eating large quantities of fat-laden cheese. Their ability to deal with the fat has been linked to their consumption of wine, and since this study, it has been judged that small quantities of alcohol can ameliorate some of the effects of eating fat. (This finding should not, however, suggest that if a little bit is good, more is better.)

The biggest single killer of people in North America is **heart disease.** It kills more people than all cancers combined, and as indicated earlier, heart disease is closely correlated with the consumption of saturated fats. The adult DRV (Daily Reference Value, p. 10) for fat is 65 grams per day for a 2000 calorie diet. More than that will generally be stored as fat. As fat deposits grow, blood vessels must be constructed to nourish them, and the heart is forced to work harder to pump blood to them. In addition, moving a heavier body puts more strain on the heart and lungs.

Not all excess fat is stored. Some is converted to cholesterol. Excess cholesterol is deposited along the walls of arteries, narrowing and hardening them. Known as **plaque,** these deposits cause even more strain to be put on the heart as it labors to pump blood through rigid vessels, which can lead to heart enlargement and blood pressure increase. The more the heart labors, the more oxygen it demands. But the **coronary arteries,** which nourish the heart, can become as narrowed and hard as any other arteries, causing the blood flow to the heart to be reduced. Demands by the heart for blood and oxygen may then be felt as pain described as **angina.** Periods of angina may or may not precede a heart attack, but the attack occurs when the heart shuts down in response to too little oxygen.

A second cause of heart attacks results directly from the formation of plaque on the artery walls. The deposited plaque causes the lining of the arteries to become rough or jagged, which may trigger the formation of **blood clots.** If a clot forms and lodges in a coronary artery, blocking it, the part of the heart fed by that artery becomes oxygen deprived. The result, again, is a shutdown of the section of the heart that can't get the oxygen it needs. Blood clots can affect organs other than the heart. A clot that lodges in the brain can cause a **stroke,** and one that lodges in a lung can cause a **pulmonary embolism.**

Fat Substitutes

Even though the negative effects of eating too much fat have been well publicized, people continue to do so because fat makes food more satisfying, providing a feeling of fullness as well as flavor and texture. Until substitutes can be found that duplicate those qualities, people will continue to eat fat. Three such substitutes have been recently developed: olestra, Simplesse, and Z-trim.

Olestra. Olestra is the generic name of the chemical compound once called sucrose polyester, a combination of the disaccharide sucrose and six fatty acids. While it has the texture of fat, it is indigestible and is not absorbed. Olestra is stable enough to use in cooking, and if substituted for fat in snack foods, such as potato chips, it can reduce the amount of fat and number of calories people consume. In early 1996, the Food and Drug Administration granted Proctor & Gamble permission to market olestra under their trade name **Olean.** Unfortunately, side effects from the consumption of olestra can include abdominal cramping, loose bowel movements, or in some people, diarrhea and malabsorption of the fat-soluble vitamins A, D, E, and K. It has been proposed that products containing olestra be enriched with these vitamins before the foods are marketed.

Simplesse. Simplesse is the trade name of a fat substitute made of protein from egg whites or milk. It too has the creamy texture of fat. Unlike olestra, it can be digested and it provides calories, although only a fraction of those provided by fat. Simplesse is not heat-stable and cannot be used in cooking. It can, however, be used in such products as ice cream and condiments.

Z-trim. Z-trim is a natural, insoluble fiber product that was developed by a United States Department of Agriculture chemist. It is made from by-products of agriculture—for example, from the hulls of grains such as rice, oats, or corn or from the bran of corn or wheat. It can also be made from the hulls of legumes such as peas or soybeans. Z-trim can be made with the consistency of fat, which means that low-fat foods made with it would feel like the high-fat foods they would replace, and eating Z-trim would add fiber to the diet as well as reducing fat. Unlike olestra, Z-trim does not appear to cause digestive upset, and although it is stable enough to be used in cooking, it cannot be used for deep frying as olestra can. It is expected to be used by commercial food preparers rather than in homes.

Despite all the negative publicity they have received, the lipids are an important part of the diet and are necessary to health. They provide immediate and stored energy and are used to make necessary body chemicals, including some hormones. In addition, lipids provide taste and texture in food. It is the overconsumption of lipids, particularly the saturated fats, that has led to health problems.

Proteins are the third category of energy nutrients. Like carbohydrates and fats, they contain carbon, hydrogen, and oxygen. They resemble the lipids in that they contain carbon and hydrogen in roughly a one to two ratio and oxygen much less abundantly, but they are unique in that they also contain nitrogen. Nitrogen is the fourth most abundant element in the human body, and its principal importance is in making protein. Proteins resemble the polysaccharides in that they are large molecules that are made of repeating subunits. Unlike the polysaccharides, however, proteins contain a variety of subunits known as **amino acids.** Amino acids resemble fatty acids to the extent that they have **carboxyl groups,** but they also contain **amino groups** on their alpha carbons. They are distinguished from one another by the rest of the molecule, which is called the **side chain** (Figure 25).

AN ALPHA AMINO ACID

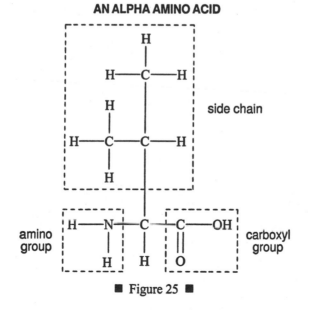

■ Figure 25 ■

There are probably many **alpha amino acids,** but only 20 occur in human protein (Figure 26). Eleven of these can be synthesized from other amino acids in human cells, but the other nine cannot. They must be eaten; consequently, they are referred to as the **essential amino acids** (labeled with * in Figure 26).

AMINO ACIDS IN HUMAN PROTEIN

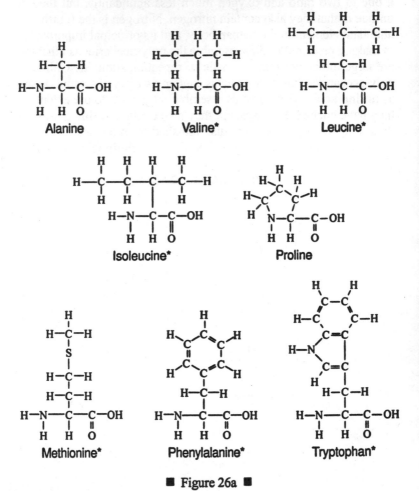

Alanine

Valine*

Leucine*

Isoleucine*

Proline

Methionine*

Phenylalanine*

Tryptophan*

■ Figure 26a ■

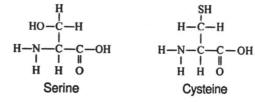

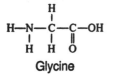

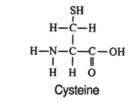

Glycine   Serine   Cysteine

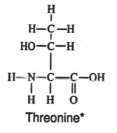

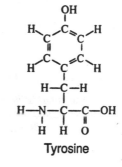

Threonine*   Tyrosine

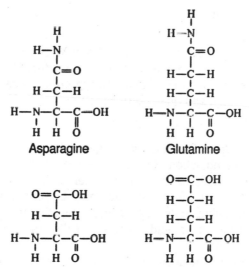

Asparagine   Glutamine

Aspartic acid   Glutamic acid

■ Figure 26b ■

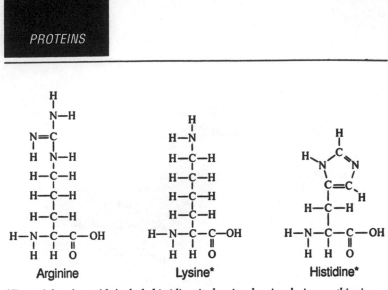

Arginine   Lysine*   Histidine*

*Essential amino acids include *histidine, isoleucine, leucine, lysine, methionine, phenylalanine, threonine, tryptophan,* and *valine.*

■ Figure 26c ■

Protein Structure

Protein plays a number of roles in the body. What role any particular protein may play is dependent upon its **structure.** There are four aspects of the structure of amino acids, appropriately named primary, secondary, tertiary, and quaternary structures.

Primary structure. Proteins are combinations of amino acids, just as words are combinations of letters. A protein may contain fewer than 100 amino acids, as in insulin, or more than 1000, as in muscle protein. Each of the 20 amino acids may be used any number of times, and the amino acids may be linked together in any order. The sequence that the amino acids assume is called the **primary structure** of the protein.

The bonding of adjacent amino acids in a protein is covalent and occurs between the carbon of the carboxyl group of one amino acid and the nitrogen of the amino group of the other. This bond is known as a **peptide bond,** and the structure formed by the two amino acids is called a **dipeptide** (Figure 27). Additional amino acids can be added to a dipeptide until a chain of amino acids, or **polypeptide,** is formed. The primary structure of the protein is the sequence of the amino acids in the polypeptide chain. All of the amino acids are bonded to one another through their carboxyl and amino groups, with their side chains extending from the line of peptide bonds.

The primary structure is critical in determining the remaining three protein structures because it is interaction among the side chains that accounts for them. If one amino acid is substituted for another, its side chain will interact with the others differently. An illustration of such a variation would be in **hemoglobin,** the oxygen-carrying protein of the blood. Hemoglobin determines the shape of the red blood cells in which it is carried. Normal red blood cells are biconcave disks. However, if one amino acid in the two polypeptide chains that make up hemoglobin is exchanged for another, the shape of the protein and that of the red blood cell change. This is essentially what happens in **sickle-cell disease,** a hereditary blood disorder in which the blood cells are crescent (sickle) shaped and unable to carry oxygen adequately.

A DIPEPTIDE

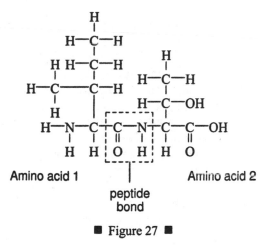

■ Figure 27 ■

Secondary, tertiary, and quaternary structures. When a polypeptide forms, it usually takes on a helical configuration, much like a corkscrew, the **secondary structure** of the protein. It results from attractive forces between the atoms in the amino and carboxyl groups. Once coiled, a protein made of many amino acids still can be extremely long. The **tertiary structure** of the protein results from the folding of the polypeptide chain, which compacts the protein. The folding results from chemical reactions among the various side chains of the amino acids, and it makes the protein somewhat globular. Finally, many proteins, for example hemoglobin, contain more than one polypeptide chain. It is the combination of these chains that makes up the **quaternary structure** of a protein. The sum of all of these structures gives each protein a unique **three-dimensional geometry.** The correct geometry is necessary if the protein is to do its job properly.

Denaturation. If the shape of a protein is altered, it is unable to carry out its function. A permanent change in the shape of a protein is called **denaturation.** Denaturation is usually the result of exposure to a physical agent such as heat or to a chemical agent such as an acid or a heavy metal.

The change that occurs in egg white when it is cooked is an example of **heat denaturation.** The prolonged exposure of body proteins to high temperature can be hazardous. For example, the irreversible brain damage that can result from a high fever may be the result of the denaturation of brain proteins. **Acid denaturation** accounts for the curdling of milk when it spoils or when one "sours" it, by adding vinegar or lemon juice to make a sour milk cake, for example. **Heavy metals** such as silver or mercury will also denature protein. Milk or egg white is often a suggested antidote to heavy-metal poisoning because the heavy metals will denature the milk or egg white protein and in the process become bound up in it, rather than denaturing the proteins of the digestive system lining or being absorbed into the blood where they can denature blood protein.

Protein Use

Tissue growth and maintenance. Protein is best known as a structural chemical; its role in muscle development is often stressed. Muscle development, however, is only one of the roles that protein plays, although certainly an important one. **Growth** is essentially the addition of tissue, and much of this process requires protein. Protein is also found in skin, hair, and organs—in fact in every cell and structure in the body. However, the need for protein does not cease when growth does. Day-to-day activities wear on the body, and protein is eroded away in the process. In fact, whole cells are lost from the skin and the lining of the digestive system by the millions each day. In order to keep the body intact, the worn tissue and lost cells must be replaced. Dietary protein provides the amino acids necessary to accomplish this body **maintenance.**

Enzymes. All of the processes that make up life are the result of innumerable chemical reactions occurring within the cells and body structures. Many of these reactions cannot occur spontaneously under conditions compatible with life (for example, adding hydrogen to oxygen to make water normally releases enough energy to cause an explosion). Other reactions, such as the breakdown of food or the synthesis of tissue, are too complicated to occur spontaneously. Specific proteins known as **enzymes** bring about these otherwise impossible reactions. Enzymes are biological **catalysts;** that is, they cause chemical reactions without being affected by them. Some enzymes are pure protein; others must contain another component, a vitamin or mineral, for example, in order to work. In the latter case, the protein component is referred to as an **apoenzyme,** and the other component is called a **coenzyme.** The chemicals on which the enzymes work are called **substrates.**

The roles of enzymes vary. Enzymes are responsible for large, general reactions, such as the digestion of food, and they catalyze the most minute reactions in the smallest components of cells. The way in which they function relates to their three-dimensional geometry.

The shape of an enzyme accommodates its substrate much as the shape of a glove accommodates a hand. The point on the enzyme at which the substrate attaches is called the **active site.** Some poisons act as protein inhibitors by occupying an enzyme's active site and not allowing the substrate entry. Others may act by denaturing the enzyme.

Hormones. Hormones, initially described on page 47, are chemical regulators that are produced in **endocrine glands.** Some hormones are made of steroids, but the majority, like insulin, are polypeptides or proteins. One, **thyroxine,** is a modified amino acid.

Antibodies. Antibodies are proteins that are produced whenever a foreign material, or **antigen,** enters the body. Many antigens are themselves proteins. They may be parts of bacteria or viruses, or they may be tissues of transplanted organs. Each antibody forms in response to a specific antigen and does its best to somehow destroy the antigen.

The presence of the antibodies in blood following the destruction of an antigen indicates ongoing protection, which is called an **immunity.** (One instance in which antibodies appear not to be protective is in HIV infection. The presence of HIV antibodies in the blood is often the first indication that a person has been exposed to the AIDS virus. The condition is described as HIV positive).

Immunities can sometimes be induced—that is, the body can be tricked into producing antibodies—by **vaccination.** Vaccines are essentially antigens that have been made harmless. When exposed to them, however, the body responds as if they were still pathogenic (capable of causing disease). Some such **artificial immunities** must be periodically renewed. Others are protective for life.

Fluid and electrolyte balance. The term **fluid,** with respect to the human body, usually refers to the various familiar liquid components of the body, such as blood, lymph, or saliva. The principal component of all body fluids is water, and the amount of water in each is critically important. Water is also a component of all nonfluid body materials, although to a much lesser extent, and again, the amount of water is critical. Proteins in cells and in spaces between cells help regulate fluid balance by absorbing and holding water. These proteins are produced by the cells and are either exported to the intercellular spaces or kept within the cell. If too much fluid gets into a cell, it can burst. Conversely, too much fluid between cells can make tissues swell, a condition referred to as **edema.**

Electrolytes are chemicals that yield ions when dissolved in water. Sometimes referred to as **salts,** these compounds, in solution, allow water to conduct an electric current. They also are involved in fluid balance; consequently, it is important that they be present in proper amounts. Two particularly important elements among the electrolytes are the minerals **sodium** and **potassium,** sodium between the cells and potassium within the cells. Carrier proteins in cell membranes transport potassium into cells and remove any sodium that has gotten in. Electrolyte deficiency can cause muscle cramping, heart irregularity, disorientation, loss of consciousness, and death.

Blood acid/base balance. Acids are compounds that release hydrogen into solution, and **bases,** or **alkalies,** absorb hydrogen. The amount of hydrogen in a solution is referred to as its **pH*.** A pH of 7 is neutral; it is neither acid nor base. A pH greater than 7 is alkaline, and a pH less than 7 is acid. Blood normally has a pH slightly greater than

---

* pH is a logarithmic measure of hydrogen ions in solution. It is determined as a comparison to how much hydrogen is in a sample of pure, distilled water. One out of every 10 million water molecules dissociates to form a hydrogen ion (H^+) and a hydroxyl ion (OH^-). The fraction 1/10,000,000 can be expressed as 10^{-7}. To express pH, only the 7 is used: pH = 7. A strong acid such as hydrochloric acid (HCl) dissociates more completely than does water. In a solution of HCl, one out of 100 molecules may dissociate, in which case the fraction would be expressed as 1/100. This can be expressed as 10^{-2}. The pH of this solution, then, would be written as pH = 2. The smaller number, 2, represents a strong acid, the larger number, 7, represents a neutral solution, and a number larger than 7 represents an alkaline solution.

7; it is very mildly alkaline. Proteins help maintain the pH of blood; that is, they **buffer** the blood by absorbing hydrogen when it is excessive and releasing hydrogen into the blood when it is deficient. Obviously there are limits to how much hydrogen a protein can donate, and there are limits to how much it can absorb. If a protein is exposed to too much hydrogen—that is, if it is subjected to a strong acid—it undergoes **acid denaturation** (see p. 92).

Calories. No other nutrient can be substituted for protein in the processes just described. However, if necessary, protein can be substituted for carbohydrates and fats to provide energy. This is not the most desirable use of protein. In fact, when protein is used for energy, it is sometimes said to be "wasted." Meeting calorie requirements is the body's most urgent need. Consequently, if too little fat and/or carbohydrate is available for use, the body turns to dietary protein to provide the missing calories. If there is too little dietary protein, the body will begin to cannibalize its own tissues in order to get protein for energy. Dieters who consume too few calories may find that some of the weight they lose comes from protein loss in addition to fat loss. Consequently, dieters should eat enough calories to spare their tissue proteins. These calories are called **protein sparing calories.**

Before proteins can be used for energy, they must first be reduced to amino acids which then undergo **deamination.** This means their amino groups are removed. The amino groups may be used to supply a nitrogen need, or they may be converted to **urea,** the waste product of protein metabolism. Urea is transported by the blood to the kidneys, where it is removed. Once deaminated, what's left of the amino acids is then oxidized like any other nutrient or converted to carbohydrate or fat. Many people do not realize that excessive protein in the diet can contribute to obesity if it provides calories beyond those that are needed. The body cannot store protein as it can fat. However, amino acids can be converted to carbohydrate (while fat cannot), which means that if sufficient carbohydrate is not present, for example to fuel the nervous system, the body will turn to protein to satisfy the need. If too little protein is provided by the diet, then body proteins will be used.

Dealing with Protein

Quality and sources of dietary protein. Proteins are not all created equal, and how a protein is used may be determined by its source. In general, proteins of highest **quality**—that is, those that best meet nutritional needs and have all of the essential amino acids in sufficient amounts—are described as **complete proteins.** Complete proteins typically come from **animal sources,** for example, dairy products, beef, poultry, and fish. These proteins are also the most easily digested and absorbed. Proteins from **legumes** (pod-forming plants like beans and peanuts) are of reasonably high quality, digestibility, and absorbability. In contrast, **grain proteins** are generally deficient in one or more essential amino acids and are described as **incomplete proteins.** These proteins are of lower quality.

Protein quality can be expressed in terms of completeness. A common measure of protein quality is the **protein digestibility-corrected amino acid score (PDCAAS).** PDCAAS scores are expressed as percentages. Complete, highest-quality proteins, such as egg white or tuna, have scores of 100%. A protein of lesser, but still good, quality, such as soybean protein, has a score in the middle 90s. A low-quality protein, such as gluten (wheat protein), has a much lower score. Another measurement of protein quality is the **protein efficiency ratio (PER).** The PER scale is concerned with protein quality in terms of supporting growth of children.

High-quality protein is critical for the maintenance of health. Tissue protein is constructed by cells by assembling amino acids that are provided by the diet. If a nonessential amino acid is missing, the cell can manufacture it, usually by fabricating it from another amino acid. However, if an essential amino acid is missing, protein synthesis stops. If the missing amino acid is not provided within a short time, the partially assembled polypeptide is disassembled, and the amino acids are either oxidized for energy or used elsewhere in the body.

The consumption of animal protein is not practiced by all people. In some cases, it's forbidden by cultural practices or it's not part of the local cuisine. Some individuals make a deliberate choice to avoid animal products. Whatever the reason, people who avoid animal products, often called **vegetarians,** may still be able to eat what amounts to complete proteins by mixing the proper incomplete proteins. This practice, called **mutual supplementation,** involves combining specific foods, each containing the essential amino acid(s) the other is missing. Usually, the foods involved are a legume and a grain. For example, in Central America, rice and black beans are used to mutually supplement one another. In Italy, this supplementation might be accomplished with pasta and garbanzo beans.

Protein digestion. Chemical digestion of protein begins in the stomach through the action of **gastric juice,** a combination of the digestive enzyme **pepsin** and **hydrochloric acid.** The pepsin breaks the protein into short chains of amino acids. The hydrochloric acid provides the acidic environment the pepsin needs, and it **denatures** the protein if cooking has not already done so. **Denaturation** is the first step in protein digestion, and cooking is the usual way this is accomplished. Heat denatures protein as well as acids do, but a protein eaten raw will be denatured by stomach acid.

There is some belief that raw protein is more easily digested and absorbed than is cooked protein, and it is not unusual to find recommendations in body-building literature to eat raw eggs. In reality, cooking protein, and thereby denaturing it, not only makes digestion easier, but also liberates other nutrients, such as iron, that accompany the protein. (Raw eggs may harbor living bacteria of the genus *Salmonella*, which causes food poisoning. Other raw proteins, such as meat and fish, may harbor living parasites or their eggs as well as bacteria.) Digestion of protein is completed in the small intestine, where the individual amino acids are liberated and absorbed. They are transported by the blood and taken up by the tissues as needed.

Protein requirements. The protein RDA varies with sex and age. For both sexes, it increases with age up to age 25, when it levels off. The RDA for men is set at 63 grams per day, and for women, who on the average are smaller than men, it is 50 grams per day. The protein RDA for pregnant women is 60 grams per day. Women nursing infants less than six months old have a protein RDA of 65 grams per day, and women nursing infants between six months and a year old have an RDA of 62 grams per day. Alternatively, protein requirement can be calculated at 0.8 grams/kg of body weight.

There are some misconceptions about protein needs. For example, some body builders, claiming that massive amounts of protein must be consumed in order to build muscle, either eat immense amounts of protein-rich food or take protein or amino acid supplements. Because protein represents the only significant source of nitrogen in the diet (p. 20), protein use can be measured as **nitrogen balance,** the difference between the amount of nitrogen consumed and the amount excreted. Growing children, pregnant women, people recovering from serious disease, and to a lesser extent, body builders are in **positive nitrogen balance.** They excrete less nitrogen than they consume, which means that they are building tissue faster than they are destroying it. Normal, healthy adults are in **nitrogen equilibrium.** The amounts of nitrogen they consume and excrete are equal. These people are building and destroying tissue at equal rates. Those in **negative nitrogen balance** excrete more nitrogen than they consume. In such people, tissue is being destroyed faster than it's being constructed, as could be the case with someone who has been confined to bed for a long time, someone who is on an excessively low-calorie diet, or an elderly person who is approaching the end of his or her life. While body builders are in positive nitrogen balance, there is usually no need for them to consume extra protein or take supplements. The American diet contains plenty of protein to accommodate their needs.

Protein excess. When massive amounts of protein are eaten in the mistaken idea that it will promote muscle growth, the majority of that protein is degraded for energy. Protein is not directly added to muscle. Rather, it is taken as needed from the dietary supply. Most

Americans eat plenty of protein, which provides more than is needed for muscle development, and the excess is wasted. Using protein for energy is expensive, since protein-based foods generally cost more per pound than do carbohydrates. In addition, long-term overconsumption of protein can have consequences to one's health. When protein is used for energy, the amino group is removed from the amino acids and converted to urea by the liver. The kidneys filter urea from the blood; however, over a lifetime, they can be damaged in the process. Animals like cats and killer whales, whose diets are almost entirely proteinaceous foods, typically die of kidney failure, and kidney disease is not unusual among humans with diets that are excessively protein rich. In addition, protein-rich, animal-derived foods, while typically rich in many vitamins and minerals, are quite poor in fiber, vitamin C, and the B vitamin folic acid (folate). Consequently, a diet too rich in proteinaceous foods may crowd out other nutrients. Furthermore, diets high in protein may promote the excretion of the minerals zinc and calcium. Rather than being beneficial, or at worst harmless, excess protein consumption can cause the deficiency of some nutrients and, in the worst case, damage health.

Protein inadequacies. It is a bitter irony that while many people in North America consume excessive amounts of protein, people in much of the rest of the world consume inadequate amounts. For years, two distinct types of dietary protein inadequacy have been recognized: marasmus and kwashiorkor. **Marasmus** is essentially total undernutrition: a person simply does not have enough to eat. Because the diet is inadequate in carbohydrates and fats as well as in protein, marasmus is referred to as **protein-energy malnutrition.** The most common victims of marasmus are young children whose bodies waste as tissue is cannibalized to meet immediate caloric needs. If such starvation is prolonged, the children experience developmental, mental, and sexual retardation. Their growth is stunted, and they are lethargic, as if to conserve what calories they have. The eventual consequence of marasmus is death, unless food is provided. However, there is a point of no return. A child who is provided food too late in the starvation sequence can still experience permanent developmental retardation. Development occurs on a set schedule, and if a particular aspect of it does not have the nutrients necessary when it is supposed to occur, it will not occur. Furthermore, if starvation continues beyond the point where the digestive system begins to deteriorate, and digestive enzymes are no longer produced, even providing food may no longer save the child.

Kwashiorkor, a term from an African language, is roughly translated as "the devil that gets the first child when the second child comes early." Among less affluent cultures, the normal means of feeding newborns and infants is by their mothers' breast-feeding. There are numerous advantages to this natural process, one of which is that nursing mothers experience reduced fertility. Unfortunately, this is not an ironclad birth-control method; lactating women can become pregnant. Among some African cultures, if a nursing mother conceives, she immediately weans the child from the breast. If the child is old enough to eat foods that are "normal" to the culture, he or she will probably survive adequately. If not, he or she is fed a watery root extract which contains little protein. While, in theory, the child is receiving adequate calories, he or she experiences protein deficiency. Consequently, development that requires protein, such as growth, muscle and brain development, and hormonal regulation, suffer. A child with kwashiorkor typically has a distended abdomen, as if his or her stomach and intestines were stuffed. This condition may result from the child's inability to produce digestive enzymes. Any food in the intestine is not digested and accumulates fluid around itself.

Recently, some nutrition scientists have disagreed about whether or not a child with kwashiorkor does, indeed, receive adequate calories. Some believe that a diet adequate in energy probably is also adequate in protein and that children with kwashiorkor are calorie malnourished as well. Whether or not this is the case, it is certain that much of the world's population is inadequately nourished. Unfortunately, much of this malnutrition is occurring in the impoverished, underdeveloped nations that are experiencing the greatest population growth rates.

Metabolic Problems with Protein

Allergies. An **allergy** is essentially an immune response to chemicals called **allergens** that are not threatening. Recall that the immune response is a reaction to an antigen, many of which are proteins. Sometimes, the immune system responds to nonantigenic proteins, which then become allergenic. For example, an infant who is fed unmodified cow's milk may not be able to accept the amount of protein it contains and may become sensitized (develop an allergy) to it. It is also possible for an infant to become sensitized to protein in formula or even breast milk. In any case, a child who cannot tolerate milk will be deprived of all of the other nutrients in milk unless he or she is placed on a fortified, artificial formula that does not contain the protein allergen.

In general, protein allergies are not common. However, one that does occur with some frequency is **gluten intolerance,** or **celiac disease. Gluten** is the protein in wheat that gives bread dough its elasticity, and some people are allergic to it, usually beginning in childhood. In people with gluten intolerance, the gluten irritates the lining of the intestine and causes chronic diarrhea, which, in turn, causes malabsorption of nutrients in general. If people with this condition eat wheat products, they experience severe intestinal cramping, weight loss, nutrient deficiency, and in the most intense cases, intestinal bleeding. Treatment for this condition is simple; one must avoid wheat products. Unfortunately, that's hard to do because wheat is used in so many foods.

Phenylketonuria. Phenylketonuria (PKU) is a problem with the essential amino acid **phenylalanine** rather than with protein in general. It is an inherited condition where one must inherit a gene for it from *both* parents. As with the inherited condition **galactosemia** (p. 56), neither parent need have PKU, but both must, at least, carry the disorder by inheriting a gene for it from only one parent. Normally, people convert excess phenylalanine to the amino acid tyrosine. However, people with PKU lack the enzyme necessary for the conversion.

During prenatal development, the amount of phenylalanine an embryo receives is regulated by its mother. After birth, when a child drinks milk, which contains phenylalanine in abundance, the compound accumulates in the child's blood, body fluids, and urine. The presence of too much phenylalanine in the cerebral fluid, which surrounds the brain, affects mental development. A child born with PKU at one time inevitably became mentally retarded. Now, however, newborns are routinely screened for the condition. When it is found, it is easily treated by putting the infant on a diet that is restricted in phenylalanine. The child then develops normally.

Phenylketonuria is not normally a problem in affected adults who have grown up on a phenylalanine-restricted diet. Most of what they eat as adults does not contain excessive phenylalanine. A possible exception is the artificial sweetener **aspartame** (NutraSweet). Aspartame is a combination of two amino acids: phenylalanine and aspartic acid. The phenylalanine is separated from the aspartic acid during digestion. Conceivably, a phenylketonuric could ingest enough aspartame for blood levels of phenylalanine to cause problems. Consequently, foods sweetened with aspartame carry a warning on their labels.

Vitamins are a collection of dissimilar organic compounds that have two characteristics in common: they are necessary in small amounts to human health, and they cannot be manufactured internally (that is, they must be consumed). They are therefore described as **essential nutrients.** An awareness of the effect of vitamins, if not their specific identification, has been around for 200 years or so, since a British physician discovered that the disease **scurvy,** which developed among sailors on extended sea voyages, could be prevented by providing the sailors with daily doses of lime juice. However, the chemical nature of vitamins has been determined only during this century. There is much misunderstanding about vitamins. Some people are under the misconception that by taking massive amounts, or **megadoses,** of vitamins, they will be guaranteed good health. Some believe vitamins are the key to unlocking reserves of energy. Others believe that megadoses of vitamins can cure anything from diabetes, to sexual dysfunction, to cancer. Others believe that while megadoses of vitamins may not be a solution to all of their health problems, they at least do no harm.

Unfortunately, none of these assumptions are correct. First, vitamins are consumed in quantities that are too small to provide any energy; only the energy nutrients do that, although they do it with the help of vitamins. Second, the only diseases that vitamins can prevent or cure are vitamin deficiencies. Finally, rather than being harmless in excess, some vitamins are toxic. Regrettably, research on vitamins to verify or refute many of the claims can be difficult. Research on vitamins is best done by **deprivation experiments** on laboratory animals, in which the animals are given carefully prepared diets that are adequate in all nutrients but the one under investigation. However, not all animals share the same list of essential nutrients as ourselves. If a specific type of laboratory animal is capable of manufacturing a vitamin internally and therefore does not require it, the animal will never develop deficiency symptoms, regardless of how long it is deprived.

Some vitamins are consumed as they are chemically used; that is, they undergo no modification internally. Others are consumed in an inactive form and are converted to their active form by internal enzymes. The inactive forms that are consumed are referred to as **provitamins** or **precursors.** A food that is rich in precursors may not contain the vitamin itself, but it is still a good source of the vitamin.

When vitamins were first discovered, they were named by letter. More recently, they are becoming identified by chemical names, although many of the alphabetical designations persist.

In general, vitamin RDAs are a factor of body size, so male RDAs for vitamins exceed female RDAs, since men, on the average, are larger than women. Similarly, adult RDAs are greater than those of children, and children's RDAs increase with growth. Pregnancy and lactation generally increase women's RDAs, and adult RDAs for some vitamins decline for individuals after age 50.

The vitamins naturally separate into two categories: the fat-soluble vitamins and the water-soluble vitamins. Their names are derived from the types of compounds in which they can be naturally dissolved, and they sometimes indicate the kinds of foods in which the vitamins may be found. Water-soluble vitamins are common in watery foods such as fruits, while fat-soluble vitamins are more abundant in fatty or oily foods such as meats or seeds, but neither is limited to any single category of foods. In general, the fat-soluble vitamins can be stored in human tissues; consequently, they can theoretically build up to potentially toxic levels if overconsumed. In contrast, the water-soluble vitamins are excreted in sweat and/or urine. Therefore, there is little worry about toxicity when the water-soluble vitamins are consumed in food. Excessive vitamin supplementation may, however, lead to problems.

The Fat-Soluble Vitamins

There are four **fat-soluble vitamins: A, D, E,** and **K.** All four are found in fatty and oily foods, and all four are capable of being stored in fatty tissues in the body. Consequently, one need not consume them every day. As long as one averages the RDA for the fat-soluble vitamins over time, one should not become deficient in any of them.

Vitamin A. Vitamin A occurs naturally in two forms: active, fat-soluble **retinol,** which is generally derived from animal tissues, and a water-soluble precursor, **provitamin A,** or as it's more commonly known, **beta carotene,** which is derived from plants and is converted to retinol by the liver once it has been consumed. Beta carotene is converted to retinol in roughly a three to one ratio; that is, three grams of beta carotene will produce approximately one gram of retinol. Retinol circulates in the blood and is selectively absorbed by cells as it is needed. The cells may then convert retinol to one of its two other active forms: **retinal** and **retinoic acid.**

The RDA for vitamin A is given in **retinol equivalents (RE),** that is the amount of active retinol the form of vitamin A provides. One RE of active retinol is approximately 0.3 µg (micrograms); one RE of beta carotene is roughly 1 µg. (A microgram is 0.000001 or 1/1,000,000 gram.) The adult male RDA for vitamin A is 1000 RE per day. The RDA for an adult female is 800 RE per day. (The designated measurement for vitamin A until fairly recently was the **international unit (IU),** and some tables still use that designation. One RE of retinol is about 3.33 IU, and one RE of beta carotene is about 10 IU.)

Vitamins A plays several roles in human health, a number of which have to do with its need by epithelial tissues (tissues that line surfaces and cavities, such as skin and the digestive lining). If vitamin A is deficient, epithelial tissues accumulate the protein **keratin,** which makes the tissues dry and brittle, a process called **keratinization.** Continued brittleness leads to cracking, which, in turn, opens the tissues to bacterial infection. Vitamin A is also important in bone growth. Bone growth is a complicated process. As new bone is added, old bone has to be removed, and vitamin A is important for that removal. Finally, vitamin A's best-known role is in vision. Part of this role is in the maintenance of the **cornea,** the clear epithelial tissue at the very front of the eye. If this tissue undergoes keratinization, it clouds. The condition can progress to **xerosis,** in which the cornea dries and thickens, and finally to **xerophthalmia,** a permanent blindness.

The more immediate role of vitamin A, however, is in the chemistry of vision. Vision results from a chemical reaction caused by light striking the **retina** of the eye. Vision depends upon the chemical **rhodopsin,** and light bleaches rhodopsin. Vitamin A is necessary for its resynthesis. An early sign of vitamin A deficiency is impaired dim-light vision, or **night blindness.**

Beta carotene is also an antioxidant and may be protective against cancer and heart disease for that reason. However, the effective form of beta carotene is that which is found in plants with numerous other compounds which may be involved with its anticancerous activities. Supplements of beta carotene have not been found to be effective in preventing cancer.

Vitamin A in its retinol form is found in foods such as liver, egg yolks, and milk and other dairy products. Beta carotene is found in dark green and yellow vegetables. Because vitamin A is a fat-soluble vitamin, it can accumulate in body tissues, but only in its retinol form. Vitamin A toxicity is not common; it can occur if a person overdoses on supplements as when a child eats a bottle of chewable vitamins because he or she likes their taste or a teenager self-medicates with vitamin A to control acne. It is also possible to toxify oneself with vitamin A by eating too much liver. In contrast, beta carotene is not toxic. It does accumulate under the skin, and if overconsumed, it can give the skin a yellow hue, but the condition is harmless, if disquieting.

Vitamin D. Vitamin D is important in calcium metabolism, specifically in the absorption of calcium in the intestine. Vitamin D deficiency in childhood causes rickets; a deficiency in adulthood causes osteomalacia. **Rickets** is a softening of the bones. Without sufficient calcium, bone cannot harden. If the bones of the legs are soft, they cannot hold the weight of the child, and they bow. If not corrected, this deficiency can cause permanent crippling. **Osteomalacia** is sometimes called **adult rickets.** Its most common victims are young women who experience calcium loss from their bones as a result of pregnancy.

The RDA for vitamin D is 10 micrograms for children beyond six months of age, young adults up to 25 years of age, and pregnant and lactating women. For adults 25 years old and over, the RDA is 5 µg. Unlike other vitamins, vitamin D need not be consumed. It can be manufactured from cholesterol in the skin by sunlight (which is why vitamin D is sometimes known as the **sunshine vitamin**). Clearly, the process is more efficient in light-skinned people than in darker-skinned people, and the most common victims of rickets are black children from northern cities. However, vitamin D can be consumed if exposure to sunlight is not practical. Vitamin D is routinely found in milk, to which it is artificially added. Irradiating milk with ultraviolet light also produces vitamin D. In addition, fish liver oils, particularly cod, and oily fish like tuna and salmon are good sources.

Vitamin D can accumulate to toxic levels in tissues, a condition called **hypervitaminosis D.** Its initial symptoms include headaches, diarrhea, and nausea. Prolonged overdosing can lead to calcium deposition in the vital organs and eventually death. Hypervitaminosis D can occur from overdosing on supplements. It cannot occur from drinking too much milk or eating too much fish, and it cannot occur from overexposure to the sun. The amount of vitamin D produced from exposure to sunlight is regulated by the body. After a specified amount is produced, the mechanism stops.

Vitamin E. Vitamin E, known also by the chemical name **tocopherol,** appears to function principally as an antioxidant by intercepting free radicals that would otherwise oxidize important compounds. In this capacity, it protects cell membranes and a number of tissues. The existence of vitamin E has been known for years, and it has been found to play a number of roles in addition to that of an antioxidant. It is necessary for normal nerve development, and it may be important in immunity too.

The RDA for vitamin E for men is 10 milligrams (mg) and for women 8 mg. However, vitamin E deficiencies are almost unheard of. The nutrient is widely distributed among a variety of foods, including whole grains and vegetable oils, it can be stored in very large amounts in human tissues, and the body may be capable of reusing the nutrient. Deficiencies have been induced in laboratory animals, but only by using specially formulated, vitamin E deficient diets. Among humans, vitamin E deficiencies are most likely secondary problems from other diseases, particularly those involving the malabsorption of fat. When vitamin E deficiency occurs in newborns, usually because birth occurred before sufficient vitamin E was transferred from the mother, the result is the rupture of red blood cells, or **hemolytic anemia.** Another result of vitamin E deficiency can be a neuromuscular disorder characterized by deterioration of muscle coordination and reflexes and impaired speech and vision. Another possible result of vitamin E deficiency is problems with the legs that are characterized by pain on walking and cramps in the calves of the legs at night. Finally, a painful, but otherwise nonthreatening condition experienced by many women has been linked to vitamin E deficiency. However, this condition, called **fibrocystic breast disease,** has also been related to excessive caffeine consumption. Fibrocystic breast disease responds as often to reduction of caffeine consumption as it does to vitamin E supplements.

Vitamin E has been credited with curing a lot of problems ranging from male pattern baldness to insufficient blood oxygen carrying capacity. But research has never been able to support these claims, nor has research ever documented clear toxicity from vitamin E excess. However, individuals taking anticoagulant medication who take large doses of vitamin E risk uncontrolled bleeding. Otherwise, no clear symptoms of vitamin E toxicity seem to exist.

Vitamin K. Vitamin K is necessary for the synthesis of **prothrombin,** a protein involved in blood clotting, as well as other such proteins. Without Vitamin K, serious blood loss could result from simple wounds.

The RDA for vitamin K increases with age up to a maximum of 80 μg in adult men and 65 μg in adult women, up to 50% of which may be synthesized by intestinal bacteria. Vitamin K is also found in leafy green vegetables, cruciferous vegetables, and liver, but it is probably the production by intestinal bacteria that makes vitamin K deficiencies rare. When they occur, it is usually in very young infants who have not had the chance to build up populations of intestinal bacteria or in individuals who have depleted their intestinal bacterial populations by use of antibiotics. Vitamin K toxicity is also uncommon. Food does not appear to deliver toxic amounts, but supplements can. Results of vitamin K toxicity can include brain damage, red blood cell destruction, and yellowing of the skin.

The Water-Soluble Vitamins

The **water-soluble vitamins** include vitamin C and the B complex, so-called because all of the B vitamins appear to work together. In general, the water-soluble vitamins are not stored in tissue. They must be consumed daily, and any excess is eliminated in urine and perspiration. This fact has given rise to the belief that there is no possibility of toxification from water-soluble vitamins, and many people have taken **megadoses,** amounts many times the RDA, in the mistaken belief that such doses of the nutrients bestow abundant benefits. However, there are risks in excessive consumption of some of the water-soluble vitamins, as will be described.

Vitamin C. The existence of **vitamin C,** chemically known as **ascorbic acid,** was suspected about 200 years ago when a British physician found that sailors on long voyages could avoid the disease scurvy by drinking citrus juice every day. Vitamin C is found in fresh fruits, which were not available to sailors on long voyages. The RDA for vitamin C is 60 mg in older teenagers and adults. The vitamin is important in the production of the protein **collagen,** which is essential for the formation of connective tissues, that is, bone, cartilage, fibrous tissue, scar tissue, and others. In addition, vitamin C enhances the function of the immune system in combating infections, particularly those of the respiratory system. Furthermore, vitamin C is important in the production of **thyroxine,** the hormone of the thyroid gland, and in the absorption of **iron** in the intestine. Finally, vitamin C is also an antioxidant, which protects tissues from the harm of free radicals.

Scurvy, the disease that results from vitamin C deficiency, is essentially the breakdown of collagen when vitamin C is absent. Its earliest symptom is usually bleeding gums. Later symptoms include poor appetite and the resulting weakness, cessation of growth, loosening and loss of teeth, and anemia. Scurvy is rare in the United States, since vitamin C is abundant in fresh fruits and vegetables and fruit juices and readily available in supplements. Those most at risk are people who do not eat properly, for example, those who exclude fresh fruits and vegetables and juices from their diets. Among these are the elderly, whose appetites are often depressed, and alcoholics. In addition, infants who are fed cow's milk, which has no vitamin C, are at risk. There is enough vitamin C in breast milk and formula milk to prevent scurvy; infants fed either are not at risk for scurvy. Stress and smoking cigarettes deplete the body of vitamin C. It is difficult to quantify the need for vitamin C generated by stress, but the RDA for cigarette smokers is 100 mg, an amount easily provided by a glass of orange juice.

Recently vitamin C has been the subject of controversy over its role in disease prevention and cure. Nobel prize-winning biochemist Linus Pauling published two books, one each on vitamin C and the common cold and vitamin C and cancer, in which he has recommended megadoses of the vitamin. The subsequent megadosing revealed that too much vitamin C causes nausea, abdominal cramping, and diarrhea. In addition, too much vitamin C in the system can cause false negatives on some medical diagnostic tests, particularly tests for sugar in blood or urine that could indicate diabetes or for blood in stools, which could indicate intestinal bleeding, signs of ulcers, intestinal polyps, or even cancer. Additional problems that are possible but not always seen with megadoses are kidney stones, acid/base balance disruption, and interference with vitamin E function. These problems result only from supplementation with vitamin C. Food does not deliver toxic doses.

The vitamin B complex. The **B vitamins** are often referred to as the **B complex** because the B vitamins generally work in concert for the release of energy from food. They function in general as coenzymes in the final series of biochemical reactions that harvest the energy in food (**Krebs cycle, electron transport,** p. 63).

Although the B vitamins are important in getting energy from food, they provide no energy of their own. Athletes who take megadoses of B vitamins in the hope of enhancing their performance do themselves no favor if they do not eat properly. If one of the B vitamins is deficient, the entire electron transport series is affected. Perhaps because all of the B vitamins work together, their deficiency symptoms are quite similar. However, dietary deficiencies in several present a characteristic set of symptoms. Some of the B vitamins are toxic in excess, although toxicity is a result of oversupplementation. Food does not deliver toxic doses of B vitamins.

Vitamin B_1—thiamin: The thiamin RDA for adult males is 1.5 mg, decreasing to 1.2 mg after age 50. For adult females it is 1.1 mg, decreasing to 1.0 mg, again after age 50. Thiamin is found in meat, whole-grain cereals, nuts, soybeans, most vegetables, and yeast.

In addition to its role in energy metabolism, thiamin is important in the functioning of the nervous system. A deficiency of this nutrient causes **beriberi,** which is characterized by progressive deterioration of nerve function: loss of sensation in the extremities, muscular weakness, and paralysis. Even permanent brain damage is possible. Heart function is also affected. Beriberi was first observed in the Orient when the practice of removing the bran from rice began. Until then, when people there ate whole-grain rice, beriberi was not known. Today thiamin deficiency can be induced by alcoholism. Alcohol causes thiamin to be lost in urine.

Vitamin B_2—riboflavin: The RDA for riboflavin reaches its maximum of 1.8 mg in males between the ages of 15 and 18. It decreases to 1.7 mg from age 19 to 50, and thereafter to 1.4 mg. The female RDA for riboflavin is 1.3 mg from age 11 on, decreasing to 1.0 mg after age 50. The vitamin is found in dairy products, leafy green vegetables, meats, and whole-grain or enriched grain products.

Riboflavin's function, in addition to energy metabolism, is to maintain normal vision and skin condition. Riboflavin deficiency is called **ariboflavinosis,** and it is characterized by cracking at the corners of the mouth, tongue discoloration, sensitivity to light, and skin rash. Riboflavin deficiency often accompanies thiamin deficiency, which may mask its presence. Because the foods that contain thiamin generally contain some riboflavin, treatment of beriberi can relieve ariboflavinosis.

Vitamin B_6—pyridoxine, pyridoxal, and pyridoxamine: Vitamin B_6 occurs in three active forms: pyridoxine, pyridoxal, and pyridoxamine. It assists in amino acid conversions and in the conversion of the essential amino acid **tryptophan** to the B vitamin **niacin** in cells. It is also important in the synthesis of hemoglobin and in releasing glucose from glycogen and has a role in immunity and the functioning of steroid hormones. The adult male RDA is 2.0 mg, and the adult female RDA is 1.6 mg. However, because of its involvement with amino acid metabolism, the B_6 requirement increases with protein consumption for both sexes, and it does not decrease after age 50. Foods that provide it include green vegetables, meats, poultry, legumes, and whole-grain cereals.

There is no name for the disease caused by vitamin B_6 deficiency, but its symptoms include skin rashes, irritability, muscle twitching, convulsions, anemia, impaired immune function, and even kidney stones. Unlike that of most of the water-soluble vitamins, vitamin B_6 excess causes clear toxicity. Doses in excess of 2.0 grams by women who were trying to relieve PMS symptoms caused numbness in extremities and sometimes in the mouth. Other symptoms included mood disorder, weakness, and walking and reflex problems.

Vitamin B_{12}—cyanocobalamin: This vitamin, with an adult RDA of 2.0 μg for both sexes, functions with the B vitamin **folic acid,** or **folate,** in the manufacture of red blood cells. Vitamin B_{12} is also necessary for the maintenance of the **myelin sheath,** the insulation surrounding nerve cells, and it may affect **osteoblasts,** cells that produce bone.

Vitamin B_{12} is found only in foods of animal origin; it is not found in the plant kingdom, and vegetarians who eat no animal material risk vitamin B_{12} deficiency, but not immediately. Enough of this vitamin to satisfy five years' needs can be stored in tissues. However, vegetarian women who are pregnant may not be able to provide enough B_{12} to their fetuses. Strict vegetarians, therefore, must take supplements of this vitamin.

There are individuals who consume adequate B_{12} but are still deficient. In order to be absorbed, vitamin B_{12} must combine with a compound produced by the stomach. The synthesis of this compound, called the **intrinsic factor,** requires a specific gene. In some people with a hereditary defect for this gene, the factor ceases to be adequately produced during middle age. Consequently, regardless of how much of the vitamin these people take, they absorb little. Without the intrinsic factor, the vitamin B_{12} deficiency disease **pernicious anemia** develops. This disease is characterized by very large immature red blood cells, damage to the myelin sheaths, and malfunctioning of the nerves and muscles.

Niacin: The maximum RDA of 20 mg for niacin occurs among males of ages 15 to 18. It drops to 19 mg between ages 19 and 50 and then drops to 15 mg. Among females, the RDA is 15 mg from age 11 to 50, after which it drops to 13 mg.

Unlike most vitamins, niacin can be made from the essential amino acid **tryptophan.** Consequently, a person who consumes adequate protein does not need niacin in the diet. Niacin promotes the health of the skin and the nervous and digestive systems and functions in releasing energy from food. Foods that provide niacin include meats, whole-grain and enriched cereals and breads, nuts, and protein-rich foods in general. However, a food that is particularly low in niacin, and in tryptophan as well, is corn. Consequently, diets high in corn but otherwise poor can cause **pellagra,** the disease that results from niacin deficiency. Pellagra is characterized by dermatitis and diarrhea initially, developing into mental degeneration and ultimately death.

In excess, niacin causes a number of symptoms, including digestive upset, dizziness and fainting, and liver malfunction. In addition, large doses of niacin can cause a sudden dilation of small blood vessels in the head, which can be painful and is perceived as a "head rush." However, some physicians are now using large doses of niacin as a medication to treat high blood cholesterol. Results have been mixed.

Folic acid: Also known as **folate** or **folacin,** this vitamin functions with vitamin B_{12} in many ways, particularly in the manufacture of blood cells. Folic acid is used in the making of new cells in general and in the synthesis of DNA. It is extremely important for fetal development (see p. 169). The RDA for folic acid for males from age 15 on is 200 µg and for females, 180 µg. It is found abundantly in liver, leafy green vegetables, legumes, and seeds. Milk may make folic acid more easily absorbed.

There are no known toxicity symptoms for overdosing, and as with vitamin B_6, the deficiency disease for folic acid does not have a name. However, because of its relationship with vitamin B_{12}, one of its deficiency symptoms is anemia. Other symptoms include digestive upset, irregularity, suppression of the immune system, and mental dysfunction. Frequent use of drugs, such as analgesics like aspirin and antacids, can interfere with folic acid metabolism. Folic acid is somewhat **heat labile,** which means that too much heat, as in cooking, destroys some of it. Therefore, raw fruits and vegetables are the best sources of folic acid.

Biotin: Biotin is a very common B vitamin that is found abundantly in foods. It is involved in energy metabolism, in amino acid metabolism, and in fat and glycogen synthesis. There are no known toxicity symptoms from excess consumption; deficiency symptoms are like those previously described for other B vitamins. These include nausea and appetite loss, depression, weakness, fatigue, and skin rashes. Information on biotin is insufficient to provide a recommended dietary allowance; therefore, the National Academy of Science has provided an **Estimated Safe and Adequate Daily Dietary Intake (ESADDI)** of this vitamin at a range of 30–100 µg.

Pantothenic acid: Another vitamin that is found abundantly in foods, pantothenic acid has an ESADDI range of 4-7 mg. Its principal role is in energy metabolism. Other than occasional cases of water retention, there appear to be no known symptoms of toxicity from excess consumption. Deficiency symptoms include intestinal upset, sleep irregularity, and fatigue.

Non-B vitamins: The non-B vitamins are three compounds, **choline, inositol,** and **lipoic acid,** that function with and like the B vitamins. However, they are not essential nutrients. They can be made internally. Choline, in fact, is the phosphate-containing component of the phospholipid lecithin. For all three of these compounds, and undoubtedly many others that play important roles in health but are not essential, the term vitamin is not appropriate, and supplementation accomplishes nothing.

Chemically, **minerals** and **water** have little in common other than that they both lack carbon, the factor that makes them inorganic. The minerals are all elements, and water is a compound. Biologically, however, minerals and water are very closely linked, and separating them, as is done for discussion in this chapter, is artificial.

The minerals can be broken into two broad categories: the **major minerals** and the **trace minerals.** The difference between the two is their abundance in the body, not their importance. The major minerals, calcium, phosphorus, potassium, sulfur, sodium, chloride, and magnesium, are present in quantities greater than 5 grams. For example, a 75 kg (approximately 165 lb) person may contain almost 1440 g (more than 3 lb) of calcium. Trace minerals are present in amounts smaller than 5 grams. In addition, there are a number of elements present in the body which may or may not have the function of minerals. In this chapter, the functions of the major minerals, trace minerals, and water are described. The major minerals are presented in order of their abundance in the body.

The Major Minerals

Calcium. Calcium is the most abundant, and perhaps the best known, of the minerals. About 99% of it is found within the bones, where it provides rigidity. However, it also plays important roles in the conduction of nerve impulses; the contraction of muscles (including the heart); the secretion of hormones, enzymes, and neurotransmitters; and the clotting of blood. The calcium needed for these functions should come from the diet, but if dietary calcium is unavailable, the body will take calcium from its own bones.

The deposition of calcium in the bones is largely a part of the growth and development process, and it is controlled by the hormone **calcitonin,** which is secreted by the thyroid gland. The bones, other than those of the skull, begin prenatally as models made of proteina-ceous cartilage; those of the skull originate as sheets of another pro-teinaceous tissue. Both undergo the process of **ossification.** In this process, crystals of **calcium phosphate** ($Ca_3[PO_4]_2$), and some **fluo-ride-containing** crystals as well, become deposited among the pro-tein fibers. The teeth form in a similar way.

The density of human bone reaches its maximum, or **peak bone mass,** at about age 30. Consequently, consumption of calcium early in life is critically important. After age 30, not much calcium is added to the bones, regardless of how much is ingested. The RDA for cal-cium for both sexes is 1200 mg from ages 11 to 24, and 800 mg thereafter. Exercise throughout life is also important to keep bones strong, but it is exercise during childhood and young adulthood that is most important in terms of depositing calcium in bones. Bones, like muscles, respond to stress by growing stronger.

Foods that provide calcium include, of course, milk and milk products, such as cottage cheese and yogurt. (Milk-fat products, such as butter or sour cream, do not provide calcium.) Other sources of calcium include oysters and canned fish, such as sardines or salmon, that are packed with their bones. Soups made from bone stocks also contain calcium. Some green vegetables, such as broccoli, mustard greens, and beet greens, are good calcium sources. However, some green vegetables contain chemicals, such as phytic acid, oxalic acid, and dietary fiber, that prevent calcium from being absorbed. Some foods become enriched with calcium during their preparation, such as canned tomatoes which have calcium-containing firming agents added. Others foods, such as calcium-fortified orange juice and high-calcium milk, have extra calcium added to them. As anyone who watches television is aware, some antacids contain calcium. Not all antacids do, however. Some contain magnesium hydroxide ($Mg[OH]_2$) or aluminum hydroxide ($Al[OH]_3$), which may exacerbate the loss of calcium.

Just consuming calcium is, however, no guarantee of adequate calcium levels in the blood. In order for calcium to be absorbed, vitamin D and fat must be present in the small intestine, along with calcium. Consequently, a person may experience the effects of cal-cium deficiency from the underconsumption of associated nutrients.

The removal of calcium from the bones is under the control of the hormone **parathormone,** which is secreted by the parathyroid glands, generally in response to low calcium levels in the blood and tissues. After age 40 or so, all people begin to experience **adult bone loss,** regardless of their calcium consumption, and consequently, experience some bone weakening as they age. The crippling condition known as **osteoporosis** occurs in those individuals in whom the bones become too fragile to support the weight of the body. Consumption of calcium after the age of 35 or so will not prevent osteoporosis; nevertheless, it may, by keeping blood and tissue calcium levels high, reduce adult bone loss. However, older people do not absorb dietary calcium as well as younger people do.

The typical victims of crippling osteoporosis are thin, elderly women of northern European ancestry. This is not to say that men and those of other ancestries are not affected, but in general, men have greater bone density than do women, and women experience an accelerated bone loss with menopause. Furthermore, people of southern European and African ancestry generally have greater bone density than do people of northern European ancestry. Osteoporosis is not well documented among Asians and Native Americans in spite of their low bone density, which leads to the supposition that genetic predisposition to the condition may be involved. Lifestyle choices can elevate osteoporosis risk. Alcoholism and cigarette smoking as well as a sedentary lifestyle contribute to bone softening.

The symptoms associated with crippling osteoporosis are generally a loss in height as the bones of the spine, that is, the vertebrae, weaken and slowly collapse on themselves. This condition results in the victim's becoming humped over and experiencing excruciating pain as the vertebrae press on spinal nerves. In severe cases of osteoporosis, the hip bone may fragment from the victim's experiencing jarring or a misstep of some sort, causing the victim to fall. Usually, medical repair of the fractured hip is impossible, and the victim is permanently confined to a wheelchair. Coincidentally, victims of osteoporosis often die within a year of suffering a crippling hip fracture.

There is no cure for osteoporosis. The only option one has is to possibly avoid it with prevention, which means ingesting adequate calcium during childhood and young adulthood, getting adequate exercise, and avoiding lifestyle choices that contribute to bone loss. Consuming adequate calcium during adulthood appears to be helpful, but it does not make up for calcium deficiency earlier in life.

The use of calcium supplements to avoid crippling from osteoporosis has become popular recently. There are a variety of supplements, two of which, **calcium carbonate** and **calcium hydroxyapatite,** interfere with the absorption of iron, may cause constipation, and, in large amounts, can form kidney stones. Calcium from so-called natural supplements, such as **bone meal, powdered bone,** or **oyster shell,** is not well absorbed, nor is calcium from **dolomite,** a form of limestone that may additionally contain toxic elements, such as lead. In general, as with most nutrients, calcium is best obtained from food.

Phosphorus. Phosphorus ranks second to calcium in abundance in the body because it is found with calcium in bone. The principal salt in bone is **calcium phosphate.** In addition, phosphorus is found in cell membranes, in DNA (deoxyribose nucleic acid), the genetic material of cells, and in ATP (adenosine triphosphate), the chemical involved in energy transfer. Phosphorus also functions in buffering the acid/base balance of cells.

The adult RDA for phosphorus for both sexes is 1200 mg up to age 24 and 800 mg thereafter; however, phosphorus is an abundant mineral in foods, and deficiency is unknown. Phosphorus is most abundant in animal tissues, but it is also found in plant materials, such as beans. Consumed in excess, phosphorus may elevate calcium excretion.

Potassium. Third in abundance in the body is the element **potassium,** the principal electrolyte found within cells. Electrolytes are elements that can conduct an electric current when dissolved in water. In the human body, they control water balance, acid/base balance, and nerve impulse transmission. Potassium functions in these phenomena, and it is necessary for protein synthesis, muscle contraction, and maintaining the regularity of the heart as well.

The estimated adult minimum daily requirement for potassium is 2000 mg. If it is not present in adequate amounts, one experiences mental confusion, muscular weakness, possible paralysis, and in extreme cases, death. Although endurance athletes, such as marathon runners, can experience muscle cramping if they lack adequate potassium, they need not imbibe sports drinks to get enough of it. Potassium is abundant in all whole foods, particularly meats, fruits, vegetables, and milk. Potassium deficiency usually results from large fluid loss, or dehydration, but it is also possible to flush potassium from the body by drinking too much water, perhaps a gallon or more a day. It is difficult to take too much potassium orally because it triggers vomiting. However, potassium introduced directly into a vein can cause death by stopping the heart.

Sulfur. Sulfur is the fourth most abundant mineral in the human body, but it cannot be classified as an essential nutrient. Because it is a component of the amino acids cystine and methionine, it is a component of virtually all of the protein we eat. In addition, it is part of the B vitamins thiamin and biotin. It is probably more accurate to describe a requirement of the nutrients that contain sulfur than it is to describe a sulfur requirement. No RDA for sulfur is given; no recommended intake is suggested. Furthermore, sulfur deficiencies are unknown. One would show symptoms of a deficiency in the nutrients that contain sulfur first.

Sodium. Sodium may be the only mineral that need not be extracted from foods. Rather, it is routinely added to food in the form of table salt, **sodium chloride** (NaCl). The importance of salt to our nutritional well-being is confirmed by its being one of the four flavors we can taste (salt, sweet, sour, and bitter). We naturally like and gravitate toward foods that have salt in them—usually prepared foods. It has been suggested that baby food manufacturers used to put salt in their products to encourage babies to eat more. Unfortunately, eating salt as an infant can cause what amounts to an addiction to salty foods, which can cause problems later in life, as described below. In the body, sodium is found principally in the fluids between cells, where it is important in maintaining fluid and electrolyte balance. It is also important in nerve impulse transmission.

The minimum daily requirement for sodium is 500 mg, an amount easily provided by most diets. In fact, the abundance of salt in prepared foods has led the National Research Council to recommend a *maximum* daily sodium intake of 2400 mg, an amount provided by six grams of salt (about a teaspoon of table salt), and one that is regularly exceeded by many Americans. The kidneys remove excess sodium from the blood and excrete it in the urine. Sodium is also lost in perspiration. After age 40 or so, the kidneys become less efficient at removing and excreting sodium. As sodium accumulates in the blood, it tends to hold water, elevating blood volume and pressure. Thus, excess sodium consumption has been linked to **hypertension,** or high blood pressure, a long-term, or *chronic*, condition. No one develops hypertension from eating an occasional bag of potato chips. In fact, any episode of abnormally high salt intake generates thirst, which is usually solved by drinking. The excess salt and water are removed together by the kidneys. Hypertension develops from a lifetime of salt overconsumption.

It is possible, although unlikely, for a person too conscientious about controlling salt intake to consume too little sodium. One reason this is unlikely is that the kidneys begin to conserve sodium if the level in the blood falls too low. A person is more likely to become depleted of sodium by a sudden fluid loss or a bout of excessive perspiration. Usually, the lost sodium can be replaced by normal eating. It is rarely necessary to resort to salt tablets to replenish the body's sodium supply. Symptoms of sodium deficiency are loss of appetite, mental apathy, and muscle cramping.

Chloride. **Chloride** is the ionic form of the element **chlorine,** and its estimated minimum requirement is 750 mg per day. Chloride is found in fluids within cells, where it accompanies potassium, and between cells, where it accompanies sodium. In fact, chloride accompanies sodium as a part of the molecule **sodium chloride,** common table salt. It is therefore found in any food that contains salt. Chloride functions in fluid and electrolyte balance, and it is also needed for the hydrochloric acid that functions in digestion in the stomach. There is some concern that chloride, rather than sodium, is the cause of hypertension among people who have chronically overconsumed salt. This connection, however, has yet to be confirmed.

Magnesium. Magnesium is the least abundant of the major minerals. It is most abundant in the bones, but about half of it is found in various organs and soft tissues. Very little is found in body fluids. The RDA is 350 mg for men and 280 mg for women. Magnesium functions in many chemical activities in the cells, including the functioning of enzymes and the metabolism of other minerals and vitamin D. It is also involved in protein synthesis and energy release.

Magnesium is part of the green plant pigment **chlorophyll** and consequently is present in any green vegetable. The darker the vegetable, like spinach, the more magnesium is probably present. However, magnesium is perhaps more abundant in seafood, nuts, whole grains, and legumes. In some parts of the United States, significant amounts may be provided by drinking water.

Poor diets may deliver inadequate amounts of magnesium. Fluid loss or alcoholism may also cause deficiency. Symptoms of magnesium deficiency include mental aberrations, such as hallucinations. They also include abnormally high cholesterol deposition in the arteries. In contrast, there are no known ill effects from overconsumption.

Trace Minerals

While present in the human body in amounts of less than 5 grams, the **trace minerals** are by no means unimportant. For example, while less than 2.5 grams of iron are normally found in a 130-pound person, iron is as important as any of the major minerals. Many of the trace minerals are present in such minute amounts that it is difficult to arrange them in order of abundance, as was done with the major minerals in this review. Furthermore, there are elements in the body whose roles as nutrients have not yet been clearly established. RDAs have been established for four trace minerals: iodine, iron, selenium, and zinc. These minerals are presented in descending order of their adult RDAs, followed by the remaining known and possible trace minerals in alphabetical order.

Zinc. **Zinc** was recognized as a nutrient in the 1960s when studies showed that it was important in the growth and maturation of children. It has since been found to be important in wound healing, taste perception, male fertility, immunity, and numerous enzyme-catalyzed reactions. In addition, it's important in the normal functioning of the digestive system.

The zinc RDA is 15 mg for men and 12 mg for women. Zinc is found in meats, seafood, whole grains, and some legumes. If zinc is deficient, not only are the functions listed above impaired, but diarrhea occurs, exacerbating the problems. Zinc absorption is inhibited by high-fiber foods such as whole grains and beans. In excess, zinc can cause problems. Too much of it can lead to dizziness and a lack of muscle coordination; anemia; nausea and vomiting; and altered cholesterol metabolism, causing accelerated atherosclerosis.

Iron. **Iron** is best known for its role in **hemoglobin,** the oxygen-carrying molecule found in red blood cells. Iron is also found in the similar compound **myoglobin,** which transports oxygen from blood into the cells of red voluntary muscle. In addition, iron is part of some of the enzymes important in releasing energy from food, and it functions in other biochemical reactions within cells.

The adult RDA for iron is 10 mg for men and 15 mg for women in their child-bearing years. After menopause, the iron RDA for women decreases to 10 mg. The reason for the higher RDA among women is the iron that must be replaced every month due to menstrual loss.

Iron deficiency is possibly the most common nutritional deficiency throughout the world, possibly because of the comparatively small amounts of animal protein that many people, particularly in poorer nations, have available to them. Red meats and liver are excellent sources of iron, as are fish and poultry. Eggs and shellfish are also good, as are legumes, dried fruits, and some dark green vegetables. Foods can become enriched with iron if they are prepared in iron cookware.

Because the absorption of iron is a complex phenomenon, simply eating iron-rich foods may not be enough to ward off iron deficiency. Much of the iron in animal protein is bound to either hemoglobin or myoglobin and is referred to as **heme iron.** Iron in animal foods which is not bound to either of the two proteins and iron from plant materials is **nonheme iron.** Of the two, heme iron is much more readily absorbed. Meat, fish, and poultry also contain a chemical known as the **MFP factor,** which enhances the absorbability of nonheme iron. The introduction of MFP factor into vegetable dishes, as, for example, by adding bacon to baked beans, enhances the absorbability of nonheme iron. Vitamin C also enhances iron absorption. Consequently, in addition to consuming enough iron, it is necessary to eat some animal foods and/or adequate vitamin C to avoid iron deficiency. Some foods contain materials that interfere with iron absorption. These include milk, coffee, tea, and whole grains. In summary, the amount of iron absorbed depends upon the form in which it is eaten and the interaction of absorption promoters and inhibitors eaten with it.

Finally, there is some daily loss of iron. As the liver breaks down old red blood cells, their hemoglobin is liberated. Most of the iron from the hemoglobin is recycled, but some of it ends up in bile and is released into the intestine. The principal way in which iron is lost, however, is from blood loss, including that resulting from menstruation.

Too little dietary iron results in iron deficiency. Its symptoms include lethargy, irritability, and, among children, short attention span. If iron deficiency becomes severe, it can affect the red blood cells and hemoglobin, reducing the blood's oxygen transporting capacity. This condition is **iron-deficiency anemia,** and its symptoms include apathy, fatigue, and chill. Iron-deficiency anemia inevitably results in energy deficiency because, once the blood becomes affected, oxygen cannot be transported to the tissues in sufficient amounts for energy to be liberated from food. In general, women are far more at risk for iron deficiency and iron-deficiency anemia than are men because of monthly menstrual blood loss and because they generally eat less. Many women rely on supplements to augment their iron intake, but there are disadvantages to that alternative. Not all supplements offer iron in an absorbable form, and some forms of supplemental iron are not well tolerated by the digestive system and cause constipation.

Excess iron can be toxic, but the risk is small. The intestines usually do not absorb much of the iron that passes through them unless there is an iron deficiency or an increased need, as in the case of pregnancy, for example. But it is possible to toxify from too much iron, a condition called **iron overload.** In most instances, this condition results from an inherited trait that makes the intestines absorb too much iron, but alcoholism can aggravate the risk. Men are more vulnerable to iron overload than are women, and the outcome can include liver damage and heart attack.

Iodine. Iodine is essential for the production of the thyroid hormone **thyroxine,** the hormone that sets the basal rate of metabolism. (Thyroxine is necessary for proper growth and development.)

The RDA for iodine is 150 μg for both sexes. If iodine is not available in sufficient quantities, the thyroid gland swells, as if simply growing larger would allow it to produce more thyroxine. This condition is called **goiter.** Iodine deficiency also causes sluggishness and weight gain. If iodine deficiency occurs during pregnancy, the fetus can suffer irreversible developmental retardation. The same severe retardation is possible if adequate iodine is not available during early childhood. This retardation, called **cretinism,** affects growth, sexual maturity, and mental development. Seafood is generally a good source of iodine. Other foods vary in their iodine content, generally reflecting the iodine content of the soils in the area where they are grown. However, most of the iodine in the American diet comes from **iodized salt,** common table salt that has been enriched with minute amounts of potassium iodide. In addition, much iodine gets into the diet through "contamination" of bakery products and milk.

Additives put in dough to preserve its texture contain iodine, and dairy equipment is disinfected with iodine-containing detergents. Iodine in large amounts is known to be poisonous. In sublethal amounts, it can cause an enlargement of the thyroid gland that resembles goiter. In infants, this enlargement can block the trachea (windpipe) and cause suffocation.

Selenium. With an RDA of 70 µg for men and 55 µg for women, **selenium** requirements are easily met by an adequate diet. In fact, selenium deficiency is difficult to cause even in laboratory animals. The deficiency is seen naturally only in areas where soil levels of selenium are low. When selenium deficiency does occur, degeneration of the heart, pancreatic damage, and muscle discomfort result.

Selenium functions as an antioxidant, which means it can sometimes be substituted for vitamin E as a scavenger for free radicals, and it may play a role in preventing cancer, although research has so far failed to demonstrate this effect. The possibility that selenium might prevent cancer has led some people to take supplements, which can lead to toxicity. Symptoms of selenium toxicity include hair loss and nail degeneration, nausea, stomach pain, diarrhea, and nerve damage. In addition to functioning as an antioxidant, selenium may have a function in thyroid hormone, though exactly what is unclear.

Boron. While the exact role of **boron** in human nutrition is not known, research has found that a deficiency of boron in the diet may have an influence on calcium metabolism and may enhance susceptibility to crippling from osteoporosis. Foods that contain boron are nuts and legumes, leafy vegetables, and fruits other than citrus.

Chromium. Chromium fuctions with the hormone **insulin** in the uptake of glucose by cells. It appears to operate as part of a complex of several organic molecules known as the **glucose tolerance factor.** Without adequate dietary chromium, insulin fails to function properly, resulting in elevated blood-glucose levels. An identical condition can occur with a diet that is high in simple sugars because such a diet depletes the body of chromium.

While there is no RDA for chromium, the National Academy of Sciences recommends a daily intake of 50 to 200 µg, a range estimated to be adequate and safe. Dietary sources of chromium include liver, nuts, and whole grains.

Cobalt. Cobalt occupies a position in the **vitamin B$_{12}$ (cyanocobalamine)** molecule that is very similar to that of iron in the hemoglobin molecule. Whether it has a separate function is unknown. No recommendation for its consumption level separate from that of vitamin B$_{12}$ is given.

Copper. Copper is important in releasing energy from food, particularly in the series of reactions in the mitochondria of cells known as **electron transport.** In addition, copper is important in the formation of some proteins, particularly collagen and hemoglobin.

The National Academy of Science's estimated safe and adequate daily intake of copper is less than 2 mg for adults. Copper deficiency is uncommon, although it can occur along with protein deficiency, iron-deficiency anemia, or zinc excess. Zinc appears to interfere with copper absorption. Copper deficiency appears to affect children particularly, causing growth and metabolic disturbance. Foods that supply copper are liver, kidneys, seafood, nuts, and seeds.

Fluoride. Fluoride is the ionic form of the element **fluorine.** Since the 1940s, it has been recognized as a protector against dental caries, or tooth decay. Whether it is an essential nutrient is yet to be determined. When fluoride is present during the formation of teeth and bones, it is taken up by these structures, which become harder as a result. Children who have grown up with fluoride available to them have generally had fewer cavities and better dental health than those who have not had it available. In fluoride-enriched drinking water, the level is generally 1 mg of fluoride per liter of water (1 part per million). Additional fluoride is obtained from food that has been processed with fluoridated water.

The National Academy of Science's recommendation for fluoride intake is a daily range of 1.5 to 4 mg. A person who drinks six glasses of fluoridated water a day would obtain the minimum amount. Where high levels of fluoride naturally exist in water, discoloration, or **fluorosis,** of the teeth may occur, the principal hazard of too much fluoride consumption. Assertions that fluoridation of drinking water poisons the water or leads to cancer are without merit, although they have been made frequently (as was, at one time, the assertion that fluoridation of drinking water was a Communist plot—also unproven).

Manganese. Daily **manganese** intake is recommended at 2 to 5 mg. The mineral functions in a number of enzyme-catalyzed reactions.

Molybdenum. Like manganese, **molybdenum** functions with enzymes. The estimated adequate and safe range for daily intake is 75 to 250 µg.

Other trace minerals. Nickel and **silicon** are known to be important in the overall health of the body. Nickel is needed for the health of the liver and other organs and tissues; silicon affects the calcification of bone.

Other minerals present in the body are **barium, cadmium, lithium, lead, mercury, silver, tin,** and **vanadium.** What roles, if any, these play is not yet determined, although lithium has been shown in many cases to stabilize the mood swings of people suffering from **manic depression.** All of the trace minerals are poisonous in excess.

Water

Life originated in **water.** Water makes up about 60% of the human body's mass. It provides an environment in which the chemical reactions that maintain life can occur. Water helps maintain body temperature by absorbing heat generated in the muscles and organs and carrying it to the body's surface where it can be radiated away. It also serves to transport nutrients and waste materials around the body. And while water provides no calories, no vitamins, and not much in minerals, no nutrient is more crucial. If one is deprived of water for three days, death occurs. The absence of no other nutrient, all foods included, kills so quickly.

Water is lost from the body constantly. It evaporates from the lungs and is carried away upon exhalation, and the body perspires continually. Perspiration increases noticeably with exercise and in elevated temperatures. Some water is lost with defecation as well. There is little control over these losses; they occur on the body's demand. The greatest water loss occurs through the kidneys by **urination. Urine formation** is very much a regulated process. Water loss through the kidneys is controlled by the **antidiuretic hormone (ADH)**, which is secreted by the posterior lobe of the pituitary gland. ADH promotes the reabsorption of water by the kidneys. Consequently, the more water one drinks, the less ADH is secreted, and the more urine is formed. Conversely, if body water volume drops too low, more ADH is secreted and less urine is formed. Low blood pressure also inhibits the secretion of ADH. Failure to produce adequate ADH results in the disease **diabetes insipidus,** which puts one at risk of dehydration from water loss by too great a production of urine. Many medications that are given to relieve high blood pressure are **diuretics;** they promote urine formation. While urine formation can be somewhat controlled, the other means of water loss cannot be, and unless that water is replaced, **dehydration** can occur. Also, urine formation cannot be totally halted, even in of the absence of water intake, because the kidneys excrete metabolic wastes, such as urea, and water is needed to carry these wastes away.

Dehydration occurs after prolonged water deprivation. As the amount of water in the body declines, blood becomes concentrated with salts, a condition recognized by the hypothalamus. In addition, the mouth and the salivary glands dry. The combination of these events is recognized as **thirst,** a desire to drink. Drinking restores moisture to the mouth and, eventually, to the blood. In general, the recommended daily consumption of water is six to eight cups. However, a diet high in salt or protein would increase water need. High-protein diets increase water need because the more protein eaten, the more urea produced. A high concentration of urea can literally burn the kidneys over time. Consequently, water is needed to dilute the urea. Salty snacks, such as potato chips, promote thirst by drawing water out of the tissues lining the mouth and by making the blood more concentrated, a condition that resembles dehydration.

The chemical quality of drinking water varies with geology. Water from regions of the world where the bedrock is largely limestone or dolomite tends to contain high levels of calcium and magnesium. Drinking such **hard water** is said to be beneficial to one's cardiovascular health. However, there are practical problems associated with hard water. It inhibits sudsing with detergents, and it causes the build-up of scale and crystals in cooking utensils and water heaters. In regions that lack limestone, the dominant mineral in the water tends to be sodium. Such water is described as **soft water.** Soft water does not leave residues on cooking utensils or in water heaters, but drinking it may contribute to heart disease and high blood pressure. Many people use water softeners, which replace the calcium and magnesium in the water that passes through them with sodium. Such devices do make the water easier to use for cleaning but do nothing to promote health. Some areas have iron, sulfur, or even natural gas in their water. These materials alter the taste of the water, but they have no known impact on health.

Recently, bottled water has become popular as an alternative to tap water. The belief that such water comes from natural sources and is therefore superior to tap water is unfounded. Unfortunately, there is no guarantee that bottled water is any more pure or free of contaminants than is regular tap water, although it often tastes better.

In summary, minerals and water are essential nutrients that do not contain carbon. Minerals and water are linked in a number of ways. The body's water balance involves interaction with minerals known as electrolytes. The water and electrolytes control the body's internal chemistry, particularly its acid/base balance. Water may help deliver some minerals to the body, and it transports them and other materials throughout the body.

One characteristic of life is a phenomenon called **homeostasis,** the tendency of a living body to regulate itself to keep everything about itself as constant as possible. For example, the normal human body temperature is 98.6°F. If that temperature begins to fall, the body shivers to generate more heat; if the body begins to overheat, perspiration cools it.

A similar regulation works in weight control. As blood sugar level drops, the **appetite control center** of the hypothalamus sends out signals recognized as **hunger,** the desire to eat. Eating elevates the blood sugar level. The appetite control center recognizes the increase in blood sugar level and signals **satiety,** the cessation of the desire to eat.

Maintaining a constant weight is, in theory, a matter of balancing the number of calories consumed (that is, energy in) with the number used (that is, energy out). In practice, it's more complicated than that. Although, over the course of a year, most people's weight changes only moderately (which suggests that weight-control regulation is generally effective), the level at which weight is maintained may not be desirable, healthy, or even normal in the statistical sense. In North America, the average weight of both sexes and among all age groups is higher than it should be. Those who are overweight are usually aware of that fact and often try to reduce weight by cutting down on the amount they eat, or **dieting.** At any moment, between 20% and 25% of U.S. men and 33% and 40% of U.S. women are actively dieting. More than $30 billion is spent every year on weight-loss plans. Unfortunately, losing unwanted weight is not as easy as simply reducing the amount one eats. This chapter considers a number of other factors that affect body weight.

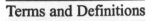

Terms and Definitions

Ideal weight. The concept of **ideal weight** centers around ranges of weights based on sex, height, and frame size. The Metropolitan Life Insurance Company determined these ranges based on the weights of people between the ages of 25 and 29 who purchased life insurance and who experienced greatest longevity. These statistics were extrapolated to the population at large. Charts showing ideal weights have been familiar sights in physicians' and high school nurses' offices for years, and the charts remain in use in many places.

There is some natural fluctuation in a person's weight over the course of a year. In general, people tend to gain some weight during colder weather and lose it in warmer weather. It is more practical to talk about an ideal range rather than an ideal weight. That range is usually given as the ideal weight plus or minus 10%. Thus, a man who is six feet tall may have an ideal weight of 160 pounds, but anything from 144 pounds to 176 pounds could be considered normal. However, if his weight falls outside the range, it has clinical implications. If an individual's weight is more than 10% under ideal weight, he or she is considered to be **underweight.** If weight exceeds ideal weight by 10% to 19%, the person is **overweight.** The condition in which weight is 20% to 49% over ideal is described as **obesity,** 50% to 99% over ideal as **super obesity,** and 100% or more over ideal as **morbid obesity.**

The idea that a precise weight range exists for everyone is appealing (and easy to grasp, which may explain why it is still often used). However, it is not completely accurate. It fails to consider that most people gain weight as they age. Consequently, ideal weight is being replaced by other guidelines, including **suggested weights** for adults from the U.S. Department of Agriculture and Department of Health and Human Services. These suggested weights present a range of weights around a midpoint and do not distinguish between the sexes (although some charts giving the ranges stipulate that the higher ends apply to men and the lower to women because of the differences in body composition). The suggested weights also allow for changes that occur with aging, giving separate ranges for adults of ages 19 to

34 and those over 34, considering weight gain and height loss that typically occur with age.

A number of factors in addition to age and sex affect weight, heredity among them. Also, being at one's theoretical ideal weight is no guarantee of health. Two individuals at their ideal weights are not equally healthy if one is lean and in shape while the other is flabby and unfit. Such individuals, one of whom may be an athelete who is "all muscle" and the other a couch potato who is not, have differences in body composition, a factor ideal weight and suggested weight tables do not consider.

Body mass index (BMI). A measure that also involves the idea of a specifically healthy weight/height relationship but also considers the relative amounts of lean and fat tissue, the **body composition** (p. 138), is the **body mass index (BMI)**. The index number is determined by dividing the square of one's height in meters into one's weight in kilograms.

$$BMI = \frac{weight\ (kg)}{height^2\ (m)}$$

The formula using English measures is similar. The difference is that the quotient must be multiplied by 705.

$$BMI = \frac{weight\ (lb)}{height^2\ (in)} \times 705$$

The BMI concept allows for the changes that occur with age. For example, the National Academy of Sciences recommends a BMI range of 19 to 24 for young adults between the ages of 19 and 24, increasing to a range of 24 to 29 for adults of age 65 and over. Because of the difference in muscle to fat ratios, men generally have slightly higher BMIs than do women.

Determination of underweight, overweight, and obesity using the BMI is grossly comparable to that using the ideal weight range. An index below the BMI range indicates underweight, while one above the range indicates overweight. Obesity is indicated by a BMI greater than 31.1 for men and greater than 32.3 for women.

The American Heart Association has recently proposed that BMI could be used in terms of ranges that coincide with health risks. The five ranges of BMIs (20–25, 25–30, 30–35, 35–40, and > 40) correspond respectively to the risk categories very low, low, moderate, high, and very high. Such terms are less subjective and less offensive than are terms like super obesity, severe obesity, or morbid obesity.

BMI is an index that considers body fat percentage in determining obesity. Consequently, other attempts to determine obesity as a factor of body fat percentage are rough estimates of BMI. A simple one is to compare the measurements of the waist and hips. A **waist to hip ratio (WHR)** of greater than 0.95 in men or 0.8 in women suggests obesity. WHR estimates central obesity, a measure of intra-abdominal fat, which can indicate a health risk, even for a person of "normal" weight.

In addition, the so-called "fat-fold" test, popularly referred to as "can you pinch an inch," provides a quick, though not clinically accurate, test for body fat content. If one can grasp an inch or more of fat, not skin or muscle, between the thumb and forefinger from the underside of the upper arm, one has a rough indication of obesity.

Body composition. The human body is composed of three major categories of materials: **lean,** or **hard, tissue; soft tissue,** or fat; and water. Lean tissue, (muscle, bone, and organs) normally makes up about 15 to 20% of total body weight, most of which is muscle. The amount of fat on the body normally ranges from 13% to 25%, and the remaining weight consists principally of water. Specific body composition varies. A man's body usually contains proportionately more muscle and less fat than a woman's. Athletes, regardless of sex, tend to have less fat and more muscle than do nonathletes. In terms of energy use, lean tissue, pound for pound, burns more calories, even at rest, than does soft tissue.

While it is generally understood that too much body fat is unhealthy, the fact that too little body fat also can be unhealthy is not. Some professional football and hockey players may reduce their body fat content to 5% or less because they need the strength and hardness muscle provides in order to take the punishment their sports involve.

In addition, since most of their energy output involves short bursts (for example, a two-minute shift on the ice for a hockey player), their principal source of fuel is usually glucose. So the reduction of body fat is not a problem in the functioning of these individuals in their sports (although it may become a problem in other circumstances). In contrast, an endurance athlete, such as a long-distance runner or a bicyclist, requires fat to fuel both muscles and heart. Athletes who don't have enough fat and who rely on glucose for an endurance event have been known to "hit the wall"; that is, they become fatigued and are unable to complete an event.

Both athletes and nonathletes use fat to some extent to insulate their bodies against cold and to protect and support some organs, such as the kidneys. Fat also provides an energy reserve. If one becomes unable to eat during, say, an illness, the fat provides the necessary energy to stay alive until eating is again possible.

Women, in particular, require a certain amount of body fat to maintain fertility. The female hormone **estrogen** is made from cholesterol, which, in turn, is made from fat. Women who drop their body fat content below their critical minimum experience **amenorrhea,** cessation of menstruation. Female athletes with low body fat content have often experienced difficulty becoming pregnant or carrying a pregnancy to term.

Such problems as these, however, are the exception. Across the United States and much of Canada, most people have to contend with the problem of too much body fat rather than too little.

The Reasons for Obesity

Energy balance. Obesity is not completely understood. It is clear that many factors affect body weight, including age, sex, diet, lifestyle, and heredity. **Energy balance** (the amount of energy consumed compared to the amount used), while not the only factor in weight control, is crucial to any discussion on obesity. Energy consumed is, of course, the number of calories that are consumed. Energy used has two components: metabolism and voluntary activity.

Metabolism is the sum of all involuntary, internal chemical activity. It includes energy spent in the normal activities of all internal organs, such as the heart, kidneys, liver, and brain, and it includes the resting energy consumption of the voluntary muscles. That part of metabolism that involves the minimum activity needed to keep a person alive for one day—that is, the amount of metabolism that would occur if one were to sleep for 24 hours—is called basal metabolism. The rate of basal metabolism is determined by the amount of thyroxine, the hormone secreted by the thyroid gland, circulating through the body and by tissue composition. Basal metabolism accounts for the largest single use of energy. On average, it consumes around 1500 calories a day. Any additional activity adds to metabolic energy consumption. In addition, added activity consumes energy on its own. The more intense the activity, the more energy consumed.

Fat-cell theory. People who are obese have at some point in their lives almost certainly experienced a positive energy balance; that is, they consumed more calories than they used—they overate. If overeating occurs at certain critical ages, specifically between 1 and 1.5 years and between 12 and 16 years, the increase in weight that ensues involves the production of new fat cells (whereas weight gained at other times usually results in already existing fat cells getting larger). A weight gain in excess of 60% of ideal weight during adulthood also generates new fat cells. Once formed, these cells remain for life, and treating obesity once these cells have formed is very difficult. This scenario has been described as the fat-cell theory. It is suggested that once these additional fat cells have formed, the body recognizes them as critical tissue. Consequently, attempts to lose weight by dieting may result in the body's attempting to conserve the cells, perhaps by becoming more efficient at absorbing the food that is eaten or by reducing metabolic rate.

In addition, the enzyme lipoprotein lipase (LPL), which is involved in the storage of fat in cells, increases as the fat cells grow in size and number, making the cells more efficient in storing fat. So those who add fat cells not only have more of them, they have more efficient ones. Therefore, in these individuals, not only is weight loss difficult, when weight is lost, LPL concentration does not change, and the lost weight is more easily regained. The role of LPL in obesity is described as the **enzyme theory of obesity.**

Weight gain in childhood that results in additional fat cells is sometimes referred to as **juvenile onset obesity.** This kind of obesity can be particularly frustrating if it is carried into adulthood because the obese adult, once having become so, may consume no more calories than does a counterpart at a healthy weight and yet remain obese.

Heredity and obesity. Studies on identical twins separated at birth have clearly demonstrated a genetic (hereditary) component of weight. In most cases, it's a hereditary tendency toward heaviness that is diet dependent; that is, a person with this tendency is not condemned to overweight, but he or she will more easily gain weight by overeating than will a person who does not have it. This tendency appears to be inherited from the maternal parent because the components of the cell that deal with energy processing, the mitochondria, are inherited only from one's mother. There is roughly a 75% chance that one's adult weight will correlate with one's mother's weight; that is, those with an overweight mother stand a 75% chance of being overweight themselves.

The **set-point theory** describes one way in which heredity may influence weight. The theory's central idea is that each body is somehow predetermined to reach a specific weight and body fat content, which it then defends by controlling eating behavior, metabolic rate, or food utilization. Individuals who fall below their set points experience some appetite elevation or absorb food more efficiently. In contrast, those whose weight climbs above their set points experience some appetite suppression or absorb food less efficiently. Since it is known that 95% of dieters who lose weight regain it within five years, the theory seems to have some merit. However, the fat-cell and enzyme theories account for this phenomenon as well as the set-point theory does.

Recent research has demonstrated the existence of a gene that dictates the production of a protein that signals satiety. Mice that lack the gene overeat and become obese because they don't realize they're full, but they lose weight when treated with the protein. It has not yet been determined that humans have a comparable gene, but the possibility that we do exists.

A critical point to remember is that heredity rarely condemns one to obesity. Instead, it can render one vulnerable to obesity if care is not taken to control eating and exercise.

Sex. Whether one is male or female also affects weight control because of variation in energy use. Since men are on average larger than women, they use more energy than women do. In addition, tissue composition of men differs from that of women. Men generally have a higher proportion of muscle, denser bones, and a lower proportion of fat than do women, even when there is no size difference. Consequently, men consume more energy in metabolism than women do. Therefore, an average-size woman who consumes as many calories as an average-size man burns fewer of those calories in metabolism and tissue maintenance and is more likely to use some of them to build fat.

Furthermore, the distribution of fat differs between the sexes. Women normally carry more fat under their skin than men do, and they carry fat on their breasts and hips, which men generally do not do. When men add body fat, they usually distribute it in the "android" or "apple" pattern; that is, they deposit it on their chests and abdomens, and more added fat may intrude among the intestines as **intra-abdominal fat.** In contrast, women usually add additional fat on the buttocks and thighs, especially before menopause. This so-called "gynoid" or "pear" pattern, is a healthier pattern than the android pattern because it does not constrict the heart or lungs. In addition, when intraabdominal fat is mobilized, it goes to the liver, where it is converted to LDL cholesterol. The frequency of obesity among women, however, is about twice that of men.

A special case exists among women who add body fat during pregnancy. Some addition of body fat is normal because of the hormonal changes that occur with pregnancy, but some women do not lose it all after delivery and may gain more with each subsequent pregnancy. On the other hand, lactation may help in shedding some of the added fat because fat is needed for milk production.

Age. People of both sexes experience increases in weight, body fat, and body mass index and a decrease in lean tissue as they age. Furthermore, women typically undergo a weight gain following menopause. It is unclear whether the gain in weight is a normal part of aging or if it is because obesity is simply becoming more common. But youth is no guarantee of leanness. In North America, obesity is now increasing among children of all ages.

Diet. The composition of food eaten, as well as the amount of food eaten, can affect obesity. Ounce for ounce, fat contains more than twice the number of calories as protein and carbohydrate, so a diet heavy in fat is more caloric than an equal-size one that is not. Furthermore, if calories are consumed as carbohydrate or protein, they must be converted to fat (since excess calories are stored as fat), and that requires some energy. In contrast, if excess calories are consumed as fat, there is no conversion and no energy consumed by it. It has been suggested that part of the increase in obesity that has been seen among children and teens is due to their having diets heavier in fat than their parents did. In addition, a diet high in fat may obligate one to eat more total food to get the carbohydrate necessary for the nervous system's energy needs.

Alcohol amounts to as much as 10% of the calories consumed by adults in the United States. Alcohol not only contains calories, but it also slows metabolism. Women tend to gain more weight due to alcohol consumption than do men. In contrast to the effects of alcohol, caffeine can increase metabolism, at least briefly.

Treating Obesity

Dieting. Technically, the term **diet** means simply what one eats. Thus, one can talk about a *balanced diet* or an *improper diet.* Popularly, however, the term has come to mean a reduced-calorie eating plan designed specifically for weight loss, and the use of such plans is the most common form of weight-loss attempt in the United States. At any time, as many as 40% of adult women and 25% of adult men are on weight-loss diets. In general, such diets do not work well. Seventy-five percent of all dieters regain lost weight within a year, and 95% regain it within five years.

Diet plans vary. Some may stress a single food or food group, others a particular eating regimen. Such **fad diets** are often based on a faulty assumption, such as that a component of a particular food will "burn" calories, whereas in reality, calories are burned by activity, either metabolic or voluntary. Some spicy foods, such as cayenne peppers, may temporarily speed up metabolism, but no food "burns" the calories in place of activity. Fad diets that stress the consumption of specific foods may be harmful in that loading up on one type of food, regardless of how nourishing it may be, can crowd out other foods that contain needed nutrients. For example, a diet that stresses fruits to the exclusion of meats and dairy products may be deficient in vitamin D or iron.

Weight-loss diets are typically low in calories and can be too low. It is popularly thought that if energy (calories) consumed is less than energy used, the difference is made up by body fat. But since fat cannot be converted to carbohydrate (the only fuel the nervous system can burn), if carbohydrate intake is deficient, the body turns to protein (which can be converted to carbohydrate). A danger of the excessively low-calorie diet is that, if the diet lacks sufficient carbohydrate or protein, the only accessible protein in the body is in critical tissue—muscles and organs—which the body cannibalizes to make the needed carbohydrate. A second danger of a diet too low in calories is that under these conditions fat is converted to ketone bodies (p. 64), which are rich in energy but toxic. In addition, a diet low in calories may also be low in essential nutrients.

In order to prevent the destruction of tissues and the build-up of toxins in response to too few calories, the body slows down its metabolism. Consequently, if a diet is to be effective, it must provide **protein sparing calories,** that is, a sufficient number of calories to prevent lean tissue destruction or ketone production.

Certain extremely low-calorie diets involve supplemental, proteinaceous drinks that contain adequate vitamins and minerals. Many of these diets are supervised by hospitals or medical clinics, where the dieter is monitored for diet-induced problems. While these diets are safer than unmonitored diets and eliminate the need to worry about vitamin or mineral deficiency, **ketosis** and metabolic slowdown still occur. The protein in the drinks is used for calories, not for tissue sparing. Tissue sparing, again, is a factor of number of calories eaten, not the amount of protein eaten. There are too few calories in the drinks for the protein to be used for anything other than energy. Furthermore, while the initial weight loss of people on these diets is often impressive, these dieters' long-term success is no better than that of dieters using other weight-loss plans.

A serious danger that has been suggested to result from dieting is called **weight cycling,** which involves losing weight, regaining it, losing it, and so on. Often the weight lost includes protein, and that regained is mostly fat. Such cycling puts a dieter at greater risk of heart disease, and weight cyclers overall have a higher death rate than do people of the same age whose weight is stable, even if they are obese. Ironically, after a series of diets, weight cyclers often end up heavier that they were at the beginning of their dieting.

Meal skipping. Perhaps falling under the broad category of dieting, skipping meals can be an attempt to reduce calorie intake. The meal that's skipped is usually breakfast, but this practice, rather than reducing calorie intake, may actually increase it by promoting overeating at other meals or between meals over the rest of the day. The later in the day calories are consumed, the more they appear to promote weight gain.

Diet pills. A variety of materials available in tablet form can be grouped under the broad category of **diet pills.** Some are simply caffeine or fiber pills, which, by themselves, don't do very much for weight loss. Others, however, are prescription drugs, such as amphetamines or hormones.

Amphetamines, known also as "pep pills" or by their street name, "speed," are supposed to effect a weight loss by accelerating metabolism. They have not been effective and have the additional disadvantage of being addictive. Those who try them have the double frustration of both not losing weight and having to deal with a drug addiction.

Medications known as **diuretics** have also been used in attempts to lose weight. Known also as "water pills," these are kidney stimulants that promote water loss by urination. One problem with using these medications for weight loss is that excess weight is not simply water. Another problem is that water lost as a result of diuretic use must be replaced by drinking or dehydration may occur.

Certain **antidepressive drugs** appear to have some effect on weight loss by increasing the circulating level of **serotonin,** a neurochemical that has appetite-reducing characteristics. **Hormones,** particularly **thyroxine,** are also thought to be effective in promoting weight loss by accelerating metabolism. However, thyroxine can elevate blood pressure, increase heart rate, and increase intestinal motility, promoting diarrhea and fluid loss.

Other materials are currently under study for safety and effectiveness, but even if some are found to be satisfactory, the obvious question is whether the weight loss they promote will remain permanent once use of the pill has been stopped.

Exercise. The two basic types of exercise are **aerobic exercise** (sustained, endurance-type exercise) and **anaerobic exercise** (strength-building exercise). Usually, aerobic exercise involves red voluntary muscle, and anaerobic exercise involves white voluntary muscle. Both are beneficial in that they consume energy and build metabolically faster lean tissue. Aerobic activity seems to be more effective for weight loss because it burns fat along with carbohydrate (while anaerobic activity burns only carbohydrate) and because low-intensity aerobic exercise can be comfortably sustained for long periods, increasing one's energy consumption.

Surprisingly, exercise alone has been found to be only moderately effective in bringing about weight loss; however, it has other advantages, which are discussed in the chapter beginning on page 151. And a lack of exercise among TV-viewing children and young teens has been implicated, along with diet, in obesity in that group.

Behavior modification. One way to reduce calorie consumption is by **behavior modification**—recognizing behaviors that lead to overeating and changing them or by changing what one eats. For example, if you normally eat bacon, fried eggs, fried potatoes, and white toast for breakfast, you modify your behavior when you change to cereal and whole-wheat toast. Similarly, if you eliminate a usual midmorning snack, you've modified your behavior.

Behavior modification can significantly decrease the number of calories consumed if a diet of largely high-fat foots is changed to one of low-fat, high-fiber foods. Fiber in the diet may work against obesity. Foods that are high in fiber are often low in calories and fat, so at times the change from a low-fiber to a high-fiber diet brings about weight loss simply because low-calorie food displaces higher-calorie food. In addition, fiber may bind some digested food and prevent its absorption. Experiments have shown that supplemental fiber can promote weight loss.

Combined treatments. A combination of calorie-intake reduction (but not below the protein-sparing level), exercise, and behavior modification is perhaps the most effective way to bring about a weight loss. The reduction in calories and added activity generate a negative energy balance, which promotes weight loss without sacrificing lean tissue. Adding the exercise increases lean tissue mass, which elevates basal metabolism and increases long-term energy consumption. Making the exercise part of a regular routine constitutes behavior modification and may prevent subsequent regain of weight. Studies have

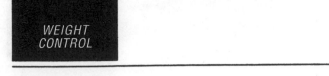

shown that such a combined approach to weight loss accomplishes more than any of the three approaches separately.

The desire of many people to lose weight supports a multibillion-dollar industry in North America. Excess weight not only detracts from appearance and sense of well-being, it also increases chances of developing heart disease, diabetes, and possibly cancer, among other diseases. While some people naturally tend toward heaviness, and an atheletic, trim body is not possible for everyone, all obese people can benefit from weight loss, even though it may be less than they desire.

Chronic Underweight

In a society in which weight loss reaches almost a religious fervor, it is not surprising that some people carry the idea to an extreme. Two behavior patterns typify the chronically underweight: anorexia and bulimia.

Anorexia nervosa. Anorexia nervosa is essentially voluntary starvation. The **anorexic** stops eating or eats so little that it essentially amounts to nothing. Typically, the victim of anorexia is an older teen or young-adult female who perceives herself to be overweight. Anorexics begin dieting to lose weight and continue on by eating less and less until they're eating practically nothing. In the process, they lose weight, but they also lose lean tissue and damage vital organs until the heart is no longer strong enough to function, even in an emaciated body.

Anorexia is a psychological problem. Anorexics have an inaccurate self-image, and the only way to treat them is with psychological intervention. Anorexics' incorrect self-image must be corrected, and they must be taught to eat again, a kind of behavior modification in reverse of that used to treat obesity. It is critical that the intervention not be delayed because there is a point of no return. If intervention is successful in treating the eating pattern but is too late, the heart can be too weakened to recover and death becomes inevitable.

Bulimia nervosa. The victims of **bulimia,** like those of anorexia, are typically young and female. Rather than starving themselves, **bulimics** indulge in episodes of binge eating, sometimes ingesting large amounts of food and then inducing vomiting to rid the body of the food just eaten. Some bulimics attempt to use laxatives to accomplish the same end, to prevent the food from being absorbed. The binge eating may occur rarely or often, depending on the severity of the disorder. The bulimic faces the same risks as does the anorexic, though bulimia can conceivably go on for years. If so, the bulimic faces additional risks that stomach acids and enzymes will damage the tissues of the esophagus and the mouth, erode the teeth, and possibly eventually cause cancer.

While maintenance of ideal weight is generally perceived as healthful and attractive, **fitness** is more often thought of as athletic capability and capacity for endurance. However, fitness is important for the health of every human being.

The American College of Sports Medicine recommends that everyone should accumulate at least 30 minutes of physical activity almost every day of the week. The recommendation is intended to help people avoid the illnesses that accompany a sedentary lifestyle. (The type of activity referred to is not necessarily vigorous exercise; it can be as simple as walking or gardening.) It is work, the challenge to the heart and muscles, that develops fitness, and whether the fitness is for the maintenance of health or the training of an athlete, it requires proper nutrition.

Terms and Definitions

Aerobic exercise. Aerobic exercise is sustained physical activity, generally enough to raise the heart rate to 100 beats per minute and keep it there for 20 minutes or longer. It particularly involves the red voluntary muscles, which, when properly conditioned, are able to carry on such sustained function without fatigue. Aerobic exercise increases blood volume and red blood cell number; consequently, the oxygen-carrying capacity of the blood increases. Such exercise involves large muscle groups, but it also involves the **intercostal muscles** of the chest, which lift the ribs and help inflate the lungs. Thus, the lungs can be filled more efficiently. In addition, aerobic exercise conditions the heart, allowing it to pump blood more efficiently, with fewer beats. A sign of good conditioning is a low resting heart rate.

Anaerobic exercise. Anaerobic exercise is short-term, high-intensity activity, such as performing a set of biceps curls with heavy dumbbells. Anaerobic exercise increases muscle mass and tone, but it does not consume oxygen as efficiently as aerobic activity and consequently causes fatigue.

Fueling Exercise

Glucose. In the chapter on weight control, low-intensity, aerobic exercise is suggested as the best way of burning fat. Fat is an important energy source for exercise, even high-intensity, athletic exercise, but the principal fuel for this kind of activity is **glucose.** Recall that glucose is stored in both the liver and the muscles as **glycogen.** Liver glycogen is used to provide for the carbohydrate needs of the body in general, and it is the source of glucose when the body is at rest.

Although less than half of the body's energy needs at rest are met by glucose, when physical activity starts, the glycogen stored in the muscles provides the additional energy needed for that activity. Unlike liver glycogen, muscle glycogen is used in the cell in which it is stored. As long as the exercise does not become too intense, muscle glycogen is used with fat as part of the fuel mixture for the functioning muscles. If the exerciser is in reasonably good shape, he or she can breathe deeply and freely enough to fully oxygenate the blood. The oxygen in the blood is delivered to the muscles, and glucose is broken down to carbon dioxide and water.

If exercise intensity increases, the muscles begin using glucose more extensively, oxygen is delivered to the muscles in less than the quantity needed, and anaerobic function kicks in. At this point, the muscles go into a condition known as **oxygen debt.** Glucose continues to be broken down to release energy, but the breakdown is incomplete, and less energy is released. A partial-breakdown product, **lactic acid,** accumulates in the muscle cells, makes them swell, and brings on fatigue. During rest, the oxygen debt is repaid. Oxygen allows the lactic acid to be broken down to carbon dioxide and water. Since some activities by their nature must be intensive and therefore fatiguing, they must be interspersed with periods of rest. (For example, a 200-meter swim sprint leaves a swimmer breathless and must be followed by a spell on the bench before another sprint can be attempted.)

Glucose is important in aerobic exercise too. For roughly the first ten minutes of an aerobic workout, glucose from muscle glycogen is the principal fuel. About 20 minutes into an exercise session, fat use becomes significant, but even so, glucose continues to be used, and the muscles take it out of the blood as well as from their own supply. Since the muscle glycogen supply can be exhausted if activity is kept up long enough, many athletes rely on high-carbohydrate drinks to supply the needed glucose for long-term activity. For endurance activities that last longer than an hour and a half, such as a marathon, athletes often take glucose during the event in the form of a sports drink or fruit juice. A high-carbohydrate meal eaten within two hours after the event tends to load the muscles with glycogen (more so than one eaten later), thus providing fuel for the next workout. As muscles become better trained, they do not burn glucose as rapidly, even at higher intensities, and they become better at using fat.

Fat. The **fat** that is used in endurance activity is principally body fat, not dietary fat. Body fat is contained both within the muscles that use it and in the fat deposits. The same fat deposits that are called upon during starvation provide the fat for sustained activity. A popular misconception is that fat provides fuel to the muscles that are close to it. Thus, it is believed that sit-ups can reduce the fat deposits on the stomach or that walking will reduce fat deposits, sometimes called cellulite, on the thighs. In reality, sit-ups are an anaerobic activity and burn glucose, not fat, and the fat used in walking comes from all over the body, not just from the legs.

The fat that's burned in exercise comes initially from the blood, where some fat freely circulates. As exercise continues, fat begins to be liberated from the fat stores, and the circulating level of fat climbs. Fat continues to fuel the activity as long as it remains aerobic. If oxygen debt occurs, fat use ceases, and the muscles rely solely on glycogen.

Dietary fat does not contribute readily to fueling exercise. In fact, an athlete who subsists on a high-fat diet runs the same risk for atherosclerosis as would anyone with such a diet. Furthermore, a high-fat diet tends to divert protein to be used as fuel in place of carbohydrate, rather than for building muscle. (In contrast, a high-carbohydrate diet suppresses the use of protein as fuel.)

Protein. Protein is the dominant component of muscle, a fact that has led to the misconception that athletes must eat a high-protein diet. Protein serves a number of purposes (pp. 93–97), only one of which is muscle construction. However, if protein is provided in excess of what is needed for all of its functions, the extra is used for energy. Consequently, those who eat high-protein diets tend to use some of the protein for energy in place of carbohydrate and not for muscle construction, which means that excess protein can even be converted to fat. Even well-conditioned athletes use protein as fuel, although less so than other people.

Muscle development is proportionate to muscle use. Exercise causes some destruction of muscle tissue, which is one reason that untrained muscles get so sore when they're taxed. During rest, the destruction that exercise causes is repaired, and some additional protein synthesis occurs. Exactly how much is determined by the muscle, not the diet. Most people consume sufficient protein to meet any added demand caused by exercise. Normal daily protein intake is recommended at 0.8 grams/kg of body weight, and an athlete's is recommended at 1.0 to 1.5 grams/kg of body weight. These amounts are easily met with a balanced diet. Supplemental proteins are not needed, and specific amino acid supplements are wasteful.

Vitamins and minerals. Because the **B complex vitamins** are known to be important in the release of energy from food, some athletes take large amounts of supplemental B vitamins in the mistaken belief that they will enjoy additional energy and enhanced performance. In fact, the B vitamins provide no energy at all. Energy is released from nutrients in proportion to what is required and as long as nutrients are available, not in proportion to the amounts of B vitamins present. Consequently, an athlete who takes massive amounts of B vitamins but neglects to eat properly ends up harming, rather than helping, his or her performance. Furthermore, excess consumption of some B vitamins, niacin in particular, can adversely affect athletic performance, even if adequate nutrients are present.

Although any athlete who eats a well-balanced diet generally obtains all of the vitamins needed, one case in which vitamin supplementation may be advisable is for athletes who must make a specific weight (such as wrestlers) and essentially fast to do so. In such a case, a single, daily multivitamin would probably satisfy all needs.

Most **minerals** are also adequately provided by a balanced diet. However, particular attention must be paid to a few minerals, most notably the **electrolytes, calcium,** and **iron.** Some amount of a number of minerals, these included, is lost in perspiration, although less so by trained athletes than by novices. (Magnesium is the exception; it appears to be lost in equal amounts by all active people.) Thus, legumes, leafy vegetables, and whole-wheat products should be included in the diet. These foods also provide B vitamins.

It is well known that **sodium** is shed with sweat, and some **potassium** may be lost this way too, especially if one exercises heavily. A low blood concentration of these minerals can lead to a number of difficulties, including muscle cramps, dizziness, and disorientation. Some people take salt tablets to prevent such problems, but a balanced diet normally provides adequate amounts of sodium and potassium. In fact, sodium is generally oversupplied by our diets. Potassium can be obtained from fruits and vegetables.

Iron is a mineral that endurance athletes, particularly female athletes, can lose to the point of deficiency. Some is lost in perspiration, some may be lost by the kidneys, and some may be lost from blood cells that are crushed as a result of high-impact exercise. In addition, developing red muscle exerts a demand for iron in order to produce **myoglobin.** Thus, the athlete or exerciser must include iron-rich foods, such as red meat, in the diet.

As the chapter on minerals points out, moderate exercise is necessary for the development of strong bones. However, overly intense exercise can actually cause bone injury, for example, stress fractures.

Additionally, women who exercise so much that their body fat drops enough to bring on amenorrhea experience low estrogen levels and loss of bone calcium. Calcium supplementation does not seem to alter this loss.

Water. Water is the most important nutrient for maintaining activity. Much water can be lost to perspiration during exercise, and if it is not replaced, **dehydration** can occur. (Dehydration is initially indicated by fatigue.)

The function of perspiration is to cool the body. As nutrients are burned to release energy, heat is also released. If the heat remained in the muscles, the enzymes needed for energy release would denature, and all activity would cease. The blood, however, absorbs the heat and carries it to the body surface, the skin, where some of the heat radiates away. The warming of the skin also stimulates the release of water by the sweat glands, and as this sweat evaporates, it cools the skin, thus allowing more heat to be shed. One of the reasons that hot, humid weather feels so oppressive is that the moisture in the air retards the evaporation of sweat, which, in turn, retards the loss of heat. In contrast, dry heat, such as is enjoyed in the southwestern United States, allows perspiration to evaporate easily. Consequently, the heat there does not feel so severe.

Water can be lost from perspiration two to four times more rapidly than it can be absorbed from the intestines. Consequently, anyone who plans on extended activity, such as a soccer game or a long-distance bicycle race, is wise to drink water before starting the activity, during the activity, and after the activity. In general, the best way of replacing fluids is by drinking water. Sports drinks that contain glucose and minerals may taste better than water, but they are absorbed no more rapidly, regardless of what's stated in their advertising. Furthermore, drinking water provides cooling. The water consumed at a temperature lower than that of the body absorbs heat from the body. Most exercisers and athletes do not need sports drinks unless they will be engaged in their activity for six or more hours.

In general, there is no perfect diet for any one type of athlete or exerciser. It is important that they consume sufficient carbohydrate, but otherwise they should plan for a diet that provides the RDAs for fiber, protein, vitamins, and minerals. No specific foods, supplements, or food categories can confer extra strength, speed, or endurance.

General Health

Few of us are athletes; consequently, one might ask why people in general should be concerned about nutrition for fitness. The answer is that everyone can benefit from exercise. Regular exercise strengthens the heart, tones the muscles, and provides numerous other health benefits. The increased use of calories promoted by exercise can reduce body fat, which, in turn, can help with weight control. That, in turn, can help control blood pressure and blood cholesterol level. In addition to controlling the overall cholesterol level, exercise reduces LDL, or "bad" cholesterol, and raises HDL, or "good" cholesterol, which protects against heart disease and stroke. Furthermore, weight control can help control noninsulin dependent diabetes. Exercise also reduces adult bone loss and improves lung function. Fitness even improves one's mental outlook, provides a feeling of vigor, accelerates wound healing, and promotes resistance to infection.

Nutrition and Disease

There are two principal categories of **disease:** infectious and degenerative. **Infectious diseases** are caused by a microorganism, usually a bacterium or virus. Most **degenerative diseases** are associated with aging. A third category of disease is **hereditary disease** (and heredity also plays a role in degenerative disease). There is no specific food or diet that can cure disease or guarantee its prevention, but a properly balanced diet can provide the overall health that helps ward off illness and disease.

The immune system. The body responds to infectious disease with an **immune response.** This response is a function of the **immune system;** it involves the cells, organs, and fluids described beginning on page 43. Since an immune response requires energy, those who are calorie malnourished, including dieters, are at risk of infection. Furthermore, because immune chemicals, the **antibodies,** are made of protein, adequate protein is as necessary as adequate calories. A complicating factor is that loss of appetite often accompanies infection, but those who do not eat cannot fight off infection effectively.

Part of disease resistance is keeping body linings, internal and external, intact to prevent entry by disease organisms. **Vitamin A** is important for this function. Too much vitamin A, however, weakens the immune system, as does too little **vitamin E, folic acid,** or **riboflavin.** Too little **vitamin B_{12}** causes changes in the immune cells and may delay the immune response. A **vitamin B_6** deficiency also weakens the immune system.

Vitamin C has been the subject of much controversy over its role in immunity, particularly in regard to respiratory infections associated with colds and flu. Many people take vitamin C supplements believing that they are protective against such infections or will make them less severe. Scientific research and the opinions of scientists are mixed on the subject. However, statistics do show slightly fewer and milder colds among those taking vitamin C. Nevertheless, as described earlier, there are a number of disadvantages to taking too much vitamin C.

Two minerals that appear to be important in immunity are **zinc** and **copper.** A deficiency of either reduces immune cell number and the immune response. Copper in excess has a negative effect on immunity. Excess zinc causes a change in immune cell characteristics that has an unknown effect on immune function.

As suggested earlier, a well-balanced diet usually provides all of the nutrients discussed here in adequate amounts. In summary, it is reasonable to say that while a proper diet cannot guarantee one's health, an improper diet can guarantee illness.

Degenerative disease. In some **degenerative diseases,** diet can clearly make a difference in onset and progress. For example, a diet high in saturated fats increases risk of atherosclerosis and thereby heart disease and stroke. Furthermore, obesity that results from a diet high in saturated fats increases risk of noninsulin dependent diabetes. High-fat diets have also been implicated in some forms of cancer, although to what extent is still to be determined.

Atherosclerosis may be aggravated by the oxidation of cholesterol, so **antioxidants** such as **vitamins A** and **C, beta carotene,** and the mineral **selenium** may be protective against the cardiovascular disease that can result from atherosclerosis. Although supplementation with **vitamin E** capsules has been found to be somewhat effective, again, the best way of obtaining nutrients is from food. Fruits and vegetables are the best sources of the vitamins, and diets high in them correlate with low frequencies of heart disease. Selenium is found in seafood and meat and in grains and vegetables if they're grown in selenium-containing soil.

High blood pressure (hypertension) is aggravated by atherosclerosis. Simply put, hypertension makes the heart work harder to push blood through narrowed arteries. Age and obesity are risk factors for hypertension, but genetic factors are involved as well. For example, African-Americans suffer from hypertension at roughly twice the rate of other Americans, perhaps for genetic reasons. On the other hand, African-Americans also have more hypertension than Africans, which suggests the involvement of an environmental factor.

Steps can be taken to reduce the risk of hypertension, among them consuming alcohol in moderate amounts only. (Moderate is defined as no more than two drinks per day.) Heavy alcohol consumption elevates blood pressure, and many alcoholics suffer from hypertension. Salt should be avoided by the hypertensive. It is well known that salt aggravates the disease; however, it is unclear whether avoiding salt will prevent hypertension. At worst, moderating salt will do no harm to the potentially hypertensive, and that is what public health professionals recommend.

Potassium and **calcium** may have a beneficial effect on hypertension. Exactly how potassium may help is unclear, but it is believed that it may function in both prevention and relief of hypertension.

Foods high in potassium–the fresh fruits and vegetables–are also low in salt. Conversely, processed foods are often low in potassium and high in salt.

The role of calcium in preventing or treating hypertension is likewise unclear, but surveys have shown that people with hypertension tend to consume less calcium than people with normal blood pressure. In addition, studies have found that people who do not have hypertension may still experience some blood pressure reduction with increased calcium in their diets.

A third nutrient that may be important is **magnesium.** Inadequate magnesium may lead to the constricting of blood vessels, thus raising blood pressure.

In general, foods that promote cardiovascular disease are also bad for blood pressure. Stimulants like caffeine can elevate blood pressure too. Steps that prevent diabetes also appear to be effective in preventing hypertension. As can diabetes, hypertension can be hereditary. People who have family histories of the problem must be particularly careful.

While diseases related to the heart and circulatory system are the most common degenerative diseases in North America, **cancer** is the most feared. Nutrition plays a role in cancer and its prevention; some foods tend to promote cancer while others may prevent it. Other factors are involved, however. Environmental carcinogens, such as asbestos, and risky behaviors, such as smoking, cannot be negated by eating properly. On the other hand, eating improperly may increase the risk.

Among the food materials that have been implicated as carcinogenic (cancer causing) are some food additives, such as **nitrites.** These are typically added to sandwich meats and hot dogs to prevent bacterial contamination. Once eaten, nitrites are converted to compounds called **nitrosamines,** which have been found to cause cancer in laboratory animals, although they were fed amounts (in relation to body weight) much greater than those normally consumed by people. Carcinogenic compounds are also in smoked foods such as bacon. Smoking is essentially a food-preserving function, but some of its by-products, like those of smoking tobacco, are carcinogenic. Another contributor to cancer, particularly lung cancer, is high fat consumption. A high-fat diet seems to promote a cancer's growth, however, rather than causing it. Alcohol appears to lead to cancers of the mouth and throat, and it damages the liver in ways that may lead to liver cancer.

Other nutrients appear to reduce the risk of cancer. Both **calcium** and **fiber** in amounts that meet recommendations appear to be effective in preventing colon cancer. The role of calcium is not clear, but it has been hypothesized that fiber, which promotes intestinal motility, helps carry carcinogens out of the body before they can do any damage. **Folic acid** functions in preventing cervical cancer by inhibiting the virus that apparently causes it, the sexually transmitted human papilloma virus. Too little folic acid allows the virus to become active. Again, the best way to obtain folic acid is from the diet, not from supplements.

Among the most exciting discoveries regarding cancer are the roles of the antioxidant nutrients, **vitamins C** and **E, beta carotene,** and the mineral **selenium.** The oxidation of chemicals within the body has been linked to a number of cancers, and the antioxidant nutrients function by becoming oxidized in place of the potentially carcinogenic chemicals. Fresh fruits and vegetables provide these nutrients in abundance, and consumption of these foods has been correlated with low cancer rates in a number of studies.

Equally exciting are discoveries that plants of the **mustard family** contain chemicals that are anticancerous. Known as the *Brassicaceae* or *Cruciferae* to botanists, these plants include the cabbages and their relatives, such as broccoli, cauliflower, and turnips, as well as mustard plants. The anticarcinogenic chemical in them is the nonnutrient **indole.** It is thought that indole somehow simulates protective mechanisms that detoxify carcinogens. Similar compounds may exist in some legumes and in potatoes.

Food safety. With potentially carcinogenic compounds like nitrites being routinely added to foods, it is reasonable to wonder why such compounds are used and what precautions are taken to guarantee food safety.

Some food additives have been used for a long time without having been found unsafe. These chemicals have been noted and listed by the FDA as **generally recognized as safe,** the so-called **GRAS list.** If a food additive on this list becomes suspect, it is reevaluated. Likewise, new compounds are evaluated by the FDA for safety.

In general, the law governing food safety stipulates that any chemical that has been found to cause cancer in laboratory animals cannot be added to food meant for human consumption. However, compounds such as saccharin and nitrites continue to be used based on a risk/benefit analysis. Their use is found to provide more good than harm. In other words, they are used in small enough amounts that their likelihood of causing cancer is less a risk than is the harm diabetics and consumers of processed meats would suffer were they not used.

The human life cycle can be divided into five unequal states: infancy, childhood, adolescence, adulthood, and senescence. Most of this review has dealt with the nutritional needs of adulthood; however, adulthood may include two special but related periods that warrant particular attention: pregnancy and lactation.

The types of nutrients needed in each of the five stages are the same, but their quantities, both relative to body size and absolute, change from stage to stage, and each stage has its own set of nutritional problems.

Infancy

Infancy is the period between birth and one year of age. In that time, a child's weight more than doubles. No other period of life is marked by such rapid growth. Growth is most rapid during the first six months, but as it slows during the second six months, activity increases.

During the rapid growth of the first half year, the best source of nutrients is either **breast milk** or **infant formula.** In terms of nutrition, infant formula is perfectly adequate, and when breast-feeding (or nursing, as it is also known) is not possible or practical, it is an entirely reasonable alternative. However, breast-feeding has an advantage in that the initial material a nursed baby receives from its mother, **colostrum,** is rich in antibodies that provide the infant with some protection against infection. In addition, some **proteins** in breast milk further stimulate the infant's immune system.

Cow's milk is not a satisfactory food for infants for several reasons. It does not contain as much vitamin C, essential fatty acids, and iron as does breast milk, and the fatty acids and iron it does contain are not as easily absorbed. Furthermore, exposure to cow's milk too early in life can trigger allergies to it that can last for life.

For the first four to six months, breast milk or formula are all that an infant needs. There's nothing gained by supplementing with other foods. Iron-fortified rice cereal can be added between four and six months, and strained fruits and vegetables can be added between five and seven months. Milk or formula by itself is no longer adequate after six months because of its poor iron content. While much of the iron the infant uses prior to six months was stored during fetal development, by six months, iron must be provided by the diet. Between six and eight months, soft protein foods, such as egg yolks, yogurt, and strained meats, can be added, and over the next two months, finely chopped meats and soft table foods can be started. By this time, babies are chewing, and foods such as toast are helpful. Between 10 and 12 months, more table foods can be introduced, and at a year, once allergies are less likely, whole eggs and cow's milk can be begun.

Recently, there has been some discussion about limiting fat in babies' diets and even not giving them milk. Neither is a particularly good idea. First, babies are still developing, and they need fat for the calories it provides and for the construction of tissue, particularly nervous tissue. Second, milk is an excellent source of calcium, amino acids, and vitamins that babies need.

Childhood

By a year of age, growth has slowed, and appetite has fallen off commensurately. However, in proportion to their sizes, **children** still require more food than adults, though less than infants.

For the remainder of the growing years, heredity exerts its influence, and children grow at their own rate. Their appetites adjust correspondingly. Children between one and two years of age are called **toddlers,** and at times, toddlers appear to go on what amounts to hunger strikes, no doubt causing their parents no small amount of concern. However, if adequate amounts of food are provided, toddlers will usually take what they need.

In addition to experiencing growth in childhood, during this period, children must learn how to conduct themselves in society and begin preparing themselves for their eventual adult functioning. Toward this end, proper nutrition is necessary to provide for the mental acuity and alertness needed for learning. One study showed that when nutrient-deficient children were given supplements, their performance on intelligence tests improved measurably, while that of a control group that did not receive supplements failed to improve.

Iron deficiency is a particularly insidious affliction because its clinical symptoms do not appear until well after a child has experienced behavioral dysfunction. Iron-deficient children tend to be intellectually lethargic, with a shortened attention span; however, not all children respond to iron deficiency with identical symptoms. Some may act irritable or hyperactive; others may act withdrawn or depressed. These symptoms disappear when iron is provided. The learning disorder **hyperactivity** and the mood disorder **depression** do not respond to iron. These clinical maladies are not related to nutrition. No food causes them and none relieves them.

It is often during childhood after age two that **eating problems** begin. Children naturally like things that taste sweet, and given the opportunity, they may crowd more nourishing foods out of their diet with sweets. This habit of substituting sugary foods for more nutritious foods can begin when children eat some breakfast cereals which, despite being enriched with vitamins, are little more than sugar.

Even children who are otherwise adequately nourished still gravitate toward sweet snacks. This, by itself, is not harmful as long as the children get adequate exercise. But children now often spend time watching television that they used to spend playing. Not only does watching television burn relatively few calories, it also invites more snacking. Obesity in children has been correlated with television watching, and such obesity may mean higher serum cholesterol and problems in adulthood.

Adolescence

Adolescence roughly corresponds to the teen years, although in some people it may begin as early as age 10 and in others as late as age 16 or older. Exactly when adolescence commences is under genetic control, but it can be delayed in malnourished teens.

The onset of adolescence corresponds with the onset of **sexual maturity,** and adolescence is the most nutrient-demanding period of life. Girls need more iron once they start menstruating, and both sexes need it for muscle development. Both boys and girls need more calcium during this period than during any other.

Parents who have forgotten their own adolescent appetites are astonished by how much their teenagers eat, particularly when they realize how much it costs. But the hardy appetite ensures that adequate energy and nutrients are present for the **adolescent growth spurt.** In girls, the growth spurt begins in the late preteens and may be over by age 12. In boys, the spurt usually doesn't begin until age 12, at the earliest, and isn't complete until age 19. Some boys may continue to grow into their early 20s. At the peak of his growth, an energetic teenage boy may require in excess of 4000 calories a day.

Another thing parents tend to forget is how busy teen life can be. Teens often have jobs, which give them more money and mobility than children enjoy. As a result, they eat away from home far more frequently than do younger children, and their food choices are not necessarily any better. Teens spend a great deal of money on fast food, some of which is extremely high in fat. One company's double hamburger sandwich with bacon, cheese, and dressing provides a full day's allotment of fat. In addition, fast food burgers are not complete nutrients. Vitamins A and C, magnesium, iron, calcium, folic acid, and fiber are often inadequate in fast foods, although other nutrients may be abundant. While it is possible for teens to get missing nutrients at other meals, provided that those are well balanced, given the pace of their lives, balanced nutrition is often difficult to accomplish. Teenagers like to snack as much as younger children do, and it sometimes takes an effort to convince them to choose an apple or banana over chocolate and cream cookies. Teens also may spend too much time in front of a television or computer or game machine.

While food may be abundant, teens in the United States today are less well nourished than their parents were, and there are indications that obesity and some decrease in growth rates are now occurring among teens. Not all of this is directly related to teen behavior only, of course. Family life has changed radically over the last few decades and all people eat away from home much more than they used to. In addition, television and other sedentary distractions have become a part of the American lifestyle. Consequently, people of all ages are less active than they once were.

The skin disorder **acne** has historically and incorrectly been related to a bad diet. Chocolate, French fries, and sugar do not cause this problem. Acne results from bacterial infection of skin pores. The bacteria apparently feed on skin secretions, and as the pores are plugged by bacterial growth, the secretions cannot escape. While heredity appears to play a role in acne, the most aggravating condition is stress. The teen years are emotionally charged to begin with. Hormonal changes affect emotions as much as they do appearance, and teen emotions can be powerful. Furthermore, as teens begin to assert their independence from their parents, as is normal, conflict develops. Pressure for good grades and getting into college only magnifies the perceived problems.

If a teen suffers from unusually severe acne, medical help is often necessary. Treatment often involves topical ointments but may require antibiotic treatment as well. Because vitamin A is necessary for skin health, there has been a misconception that vitamin A supplementation can be used as an acne treatment (in fact, a topical medication exists that is made from vitamin A), but taking supplements gains nothing and can lead to problems, as vitamin A is toxic in excess. Often, the only cure for acne is to outgrow it.

Pregnancy and Lactation

Pregnancy. Pregnancy is a singular time in a woman's life. Virtually everyone advises her to watch her diet, often with the admonition "You're eating for two." While opinions on how much weight a woman should gain during pregnancy have changed over the years, there is no doubt that proper nutrition during pregnancy is vital and that both undernutrition and overnutrition can have disastrous consequences. In general, the greater a woman's body mass index, the less weight she is advised to gain during pregnancy. Most of the weight gained with pregnancy is tissue related directly to the nurturance and development of the infant, but some fat is gained to fuel lactation. Too much gain in fat, of course, is not healthy because it will be retained after delivery.

Pregnancy increases the need for most nutrients, but not all. Vitamin A and D requirements, for example, do not change. In contrast, the **iron** requirement doubles, and the **folic acid** requirement more than doubles. Other nutrient requirements also increase, but in smaller proportions. The **calorie** requirement increases too, but only by 15% or less. Consequently, nutrient-dense foods best serve a pregnant woman's needs. **Protein** needs increase by a third or less, and **fat** requirements increase as well. The growing fetus requires protein for tissue construction and fat, particularly **omega-3** and **omega-6 fatty acids,** for development of the nervous system.

Adequate nutrition during pregnancy is important to both mother and child. The bone minerals—**calcium, phosphorus,** and **magnesium**—are taken from the mother's reserves toward the end of pregnancy when the fetal bones begin to calcify. Intestinal absorption of these minerals increases early in pregnancy, thus allowing reserves to be built up. If those reserves are not built up, however, the mother's bones will be sacrificed for those of the fetus. The effects of that depletion may not show up until late in the mother's life, when she develops osteoporosis.

Inadequate nutrition may also lead to a **low-birthweight** baby, one that weighs less than 5.5 pounds. Such babies may be too weak to feed properly and, indeed, be too weak to cry loudly when hungry. In addition, low-birthweight babies have much higher death rates than do babies of normal birthweight, as much as 40 times higher.

One B vitamin, **folic acid,** is crucial for proper development of the nervous system. Without an adequate supply, nervous system disorders know as **neural tube defects** can occur. The neural tube is a developmental structure from which the central nervous system is generated. In normal infants, it becomes completely enclosed by the bones of the spinal column. However, inadequate folic acid may lead to openings left in the spinal bones through which the spinal cord can protrude. A severe case of this disorder is known as **spina bifida.**

Another problem that can develop from lack of folic acid is that the infant's brain may not develop at all, a condition called **anencephaly.** If a woman enters pregnancy folic-acid deficient, it may be too late to avoid neural tube defects.

Yet another possible consequence of inadequate nourishment during pregnancy is that the **placenta,** the structure that attaches the fetus to the wall of its mother's uterus, may fail to develop properly. All nutrients the fetus receives and all wastes it produces must cross the placenta. If it is improperly developed, the infant may develop abnormally or even die. Nutrient supplementation during pregnancy is often necessary to avoid these problems, but as always, supplementation should be undertaken only with the advice of a physician.

A nutritional complication that occasionally develops during pregnancy is **gestational diabetes.** Like other forms of diabetes, this disease involves abnormal metabolism of glucose. It is usually a temporary condition that disappears once pregnancy is over; however, if not properly managed, the condition can be serious, possibly causing the death of the fetus, the mother, or both. If this problem occurs, it is best treated by strict diet.

Morning sickness, the nausea that occurs early in pregnancy (any time of day, despite its name), results from hormonal changes. If it is debilitating, medical help may be necessary.

An often comical side effect of pregnancy is odd **food cravings.** Stories of women craving pickles and ice cream or milkshakes of weird flavors are legion. The cravings have no known nutritional basis, but that fact doesn't make them any less real to the craver. Most likely, they result from alterations in taste and smell that are caused by internal chemical changes. In nutrient-deficient pregnant women, however, a very serious condition called **pica** may occur. In this disorder, women crave nonnutrient materials, such as clay or ice. Pica is coincidental with poor nutrition; however, a clear cause-and-effect relationship has not been verified.

Lactation. Among the hormonal changes that occur during pregnancy is production and secretion of the hormone **prolactin.** This hormone promotes **lactation,** the production of milk. Like pregnancy, **breast-feeding** makes nutrient demands on the mother. In fact, the nutrient demands for lactation, other than for iron and folic acid, exceed those for pregnancy. Energy needs during lactation increase by 650 calories, on average, more than twice their increase during pregnancy. Perhaps 150 of these calories should be met by fat that was gained during pregnancy, but the remainder should be met from the diet.

Breast milk volume is determined by the demands of the infant. On average, that's about three cups per day. To meet this and all other fluid needs, it is recommended that lactating women drink at least two quarts of fluids each day. These fluids should not include beer or any other alcoholic beverage, regardless of the myth that alcohol stimulates milk production. In fact, it does not, and the alcohol may enter the mother's milk and, in turn, be transferred to the infant.

Many things a breast-feeding mother eats can end up in her milk. If the mother has too much coffee, she may make the infant nervous and wakeful. If she eats such things as onions and peanut butter, the infant may become gassy. Of course, if food chemicals a mother consumes can be transmitted to her infant, so can other things she ingests, such as drugs.

From the infant's viewpoint, breast milk is the ideal food. Infant formula, while adequate, is not better. The principal protein in milk, **alpha-lactalbumin,** is easily handled by the infant's digestive system. Another protein, **lactoferrin,** promotes the absorption of iron by the infant's digestive system, and it helps control intestinal bacteria. Vitamins and minerals are adequate in breast milk, although dark-skinned infants in northern, cloudy climates may be at risk for vitamin

D deficiency. For this reason, pediatricians recommend that vitamin D supplements be given to breast-fed infants. In addition, it is recommended that breast-fed infants begin eating an iron-fortified cereal at four months or so. Furthermore, as described on page 163, breast milk helps protect the infant from infection.

From the mother's point of view, there are advantages to nursing as well. Women at risk of breast cancer, particularly daughters of women who have had the disease, can reduce their risk by nursing their infants. The idea that mother's milk can be too rich and can cause colic in the infant or that a healthy, young woman is incapable of producing enough milk are patently false.

Senescence

Known by euphemisms like the "golden age" or "senior citizenry," **senescence** simply means older age. Everyone who lives long enough goes through it, and it presents its own challenges in terms of nutrition, particularly now that people are living longer than at any time in history. This longevity is largely a product of better medical services and improvements in hygiene. No known supplement or diet, other than eating sensibly to begin with, can prolong life, regardless of stories to the contrary. The biggest nutrition-related problem of the elderly is that many of them don't eat properly.

Bodily changes as we age are inevitable. All of our senses decline in acuity, including our senses of taste and smell. Consequently, food often becomes less appealing to older adults, a condition that may lead to **malnutrition. Protein** and **carbohydrates** continue to be important during the senior years, particularly whole-grain carbohydrates to provide fiber. **Constipation** is a common complaint among older adults, and fiber helps combat it.

Fats, on the other hand, should be restricted, not only because of their roles in heart disease, cancer, and other ailments, but because they aggravate **arthritis** as well. **Omega-6 unsaturated fatty acids,** in particular, may make the pain of arthritis worse, while **omega-3 unsaturated fatty acids,** in contrast, may relieve it. An additional reason to restrict fat is that energy needs decline starting at about age 50. Consequently, if calorie intake isn't reduced, weight gain becomes inevitable.

Vitamins, minerals, and **water,** of course, also continue to be important for seniors. The RDAs for **thiamin, riboflavin,** and **niacin,** and, for women, **iron** do decline somewhat after age 50, but those of most of the other vitamins and minerals do not. Getting enough of some of the vitamins may become difficult for older people, however. Milk and vegetable consumption decline with age, perhaps due to changing tastes, as does consumption of whole grains. So the vitamins contained within these foods are not consumed. **Zinc** deficiency can aggravate all nutritional problems because it leads to appetite depression. **Calcium** intake may also decline, again due to the consumption of less milk. **Dehydration** is also a risk as older kidneys do not reabsorb water as well as younger ones do, and many seniors do not drink enough

Recently, nutrient supplements specifically aimed at older people have come on the market. Some anecdotal evidence indicates that they are beneficial; however, there's little reason to believe that a well-balanced multivitamin and mineral pill would not do as well. Before older adults begin experimenting with either, they should consult a physician.

Senescence is simply a stage of life. In that regard, it is like any other stage, and with proper nourishment, an older adult should be able to live up to his or her potential.

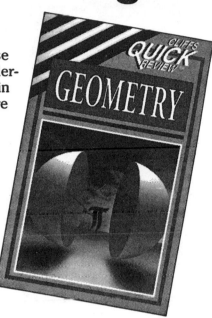
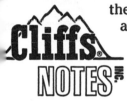

Study Smart with Cliffs StudyWare®

Cliffs StudyWare is interactive software that helps you make the most of your study time. The programs are easy to use and designed to let you work at your own pace.

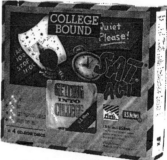

Test Preparation Guides—
Prepare for major qualifying exams. • Pinpoint strengths and weaknesses through individualized study plan. • Learn more through complete answer explanations. • Hone your skills with full-length practice tests. • Score higher by utilizing proven test-taking strategies.

Course Reviews—Designed for introductory college level courses. • Supplement class lectures and textbook reading. • Review for midterms and finals.

ty.	Title		Price	Total	Qty.	Title		Price	Total
	Algebra I	☐IBM ☐Mac	19.98			Science Bndl. (Biol., Chem., Physics)		34.98	
	Algebra I CD-ROM (IBM & Mac)		19.98			Statistics	☐IRM ☐Mac	19.98	
	Biology	☐IBM	19.98			Trigonometry (TMV)	☐IBM ☐Mac	19.98	
	Biology CD-ROM (IBM & Mac)		19.98			ACT	☐IBM ☐Mac	19.98	
	Calculus	☐IBM ☐Mac	19.98			ACT CD-ROM (IBM & Mac)		19.98	
	Calculus CD-ROM (IBM & Mac)		19.98			CBEST	☐IBM ☐Mac	19.98	
	Chemistry	☐IBM ☐Mac	19.98			College Bound Bndl. (ACT, SAT, U.S. News)		29.98	
	Chemistry CD-ROM (IBM & Mac)		19.98			GED	☐IBM ☐Mac	19.98	
	Economics	☐IBM ☐Mac	19.98			GRE	☐IBM ☐Mac	19.98	
	Geometry	☐IBM ☐Mac	19.98			GRE CD-ROM (IBM & Mac)		19.98	
	Geometry CD-ROM (IBM & Mac)		19.98			LSAT	☐IBM ☐Mac	19.98	
	Math Bundle (Alg., Calc., Geom., Trig.)		39.98			SAT I	☐IBM ☐Mac	19.98	
	Physics	☐IBM ☐Mac	19.98			SAT I CD-ROM (IBM & Mac)		19.98	

Prices subject to change without notice.

ilable at your ksellers, or send form with your ck or money order to s Notes, Inc., P.O. Box 28, Lincoln, NE 68501 ://www.cliffs.com

☐ Money order   ☐ Check payable to Cliffs Notes, Inc.

☐ Visa ☐ Mastercard   Signature _____

Card no. _____ Exp. date _____

Name _____

Address _____

City _____ State_____ Zip_____

GRE is a registered trademark of ETS. SAT is a registered trademark of CEEB.

1997